MIND MIRROR

Three Minutes Without Air
Three Days Without Water
Three Weeks Without Food

By Christa A. Tullis

This book is not intended as a substitute for the medical advice of
physicians. The reader should consult a physician in matters relating
to his/her mental and physical health, particularly with respect to any
symptoms that may require diagnosis or medical attention.

Cover image provided by : Aleksandar Mijatovic/Shutterstock

Author photo by David Burt: www.davidburtimages.com

Be careful about reading health books. You may die of a misprint.
Mark Twain

DEDICATION

In loving memory of
Jipsy Janice Nufer 1913 - 2012
Royce Deryl Edwards Jr. 1971 - 2012
Anthony J Plati Jr. "Skip" 1957 - 2012
Timothy Butcher 1967 - 2012

Any man's death diminishes me, because I am involved in mankind,
and therefore never send to know for whom the bell tolls; it tolls for thee.
John Donne

TABLE OF CONTENTS

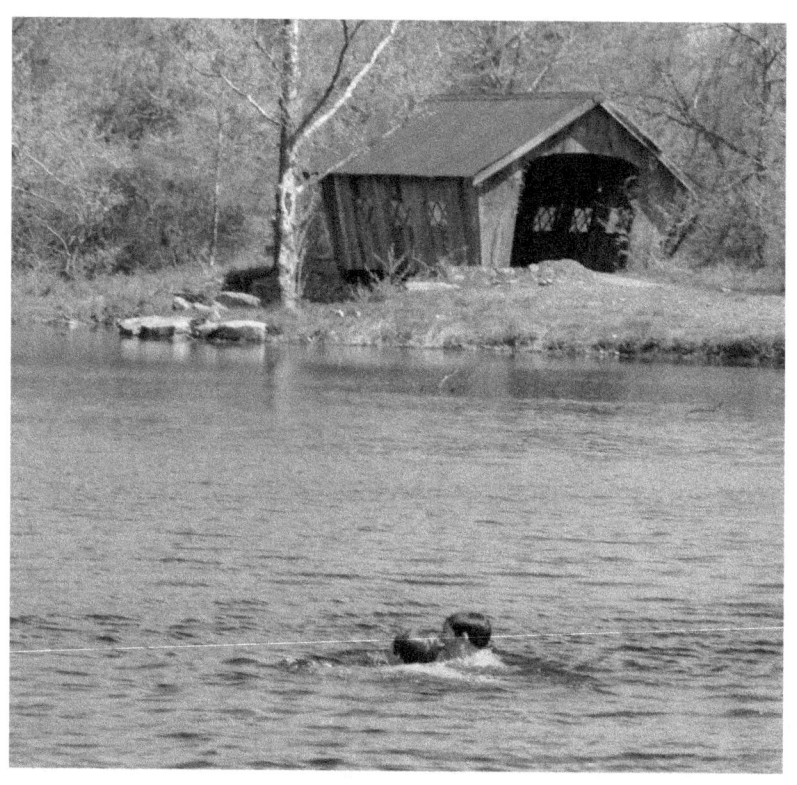

You are a child of the universe, no less than the trees and the stars; you have a right to be here. And whether or not it is clear to you, no doubt the universe is unfolding as it should. Therefore be at peace with God, whatever you conceive Him to be, and whatever your labors and aspirations, in the noisy confusion of life keep peace with your soul. With all its sham, drudgery, and broken dreams, it is still a beautiful world. Be cheerful. Strive to be happy.

Max Ehrmann *Desiderata*

PREFACE

As you simplify your life, the laws of the universe
will be simpler; solitude will not be solitude, poverty
will not be poverty, nor weakness weakness.
Henry David Thoreau

When I was a child, I never considered my body as being separate from my mind. My days were spent exploring nature and I didn't give much thought to being separate from the streams in which I swam. I was raised with six brothers and sisters on 100 acres of land. We had trees, ponds, animals, lots of freedom and I don't recall ever saying the words, *I'm bored.* As a child, I had a coyote for a pet. I would ride my horse, collecting herbs, pretending to be a medicine woman. My parents and siblings were my teachers and nature was my classroom.

Even for the 1970's, my childhood was unconventional compared to my friends. From the time I entered primary school, my mother sent notes saying for *religious reasons* I was not to have vaccinations. One day when I was old enough to understand, I asked her what the note meant and she replied, "The body is able to heal itself." It wasn't a religious reason but no one ever inquired so she used the same excuse year after year. She didn't allow the removal of my tonsils because the tonsils were the first line of defense in the body. If they were infected that meant they were doing their job of preventing bacteria from moving deeper into the body. Her goal was to prevent the problem, not eliminate the consequence. Thankfully, we had a doctor that supported my mom's decisions.

The doctor who delivered most of my mom's children continued to care for us until he was in his 80's. He was our "family" doctor in every sense of the word. Every member of our family saw him and we considered him family. His doctor's office was behind his house and had birds flying around the waiting room. Occasionally, a cat would sneak in between your legs when you walked through the door. Rarely did he prescribe any medicine when I saw him and I was never sent for *more testing*. Usually he would attribute my condition to something simple, give me an orthopedic adjustment and send me home with suggestions. He was nonchalant and not prone to making people worry unnecessarily.

To be quite honest, as a child, I usually started feeling better in the waiting room and I would pretend I was sick by the time it was my turn to see him. Later in life, I read about the *waiting room effect* in *Peace, Love and Healing* (Siegel, 1989). Your body reaches a state of healing because of the positive belief that you are getting ready to be healed. To our dismay, we don't invest enough belief in our power to heal and we end up paying dearly through exorbitant health care costs. We didn't have health insurance when I was a child. Thankfully, our doctor let my mom work in the office periodically to reimburse him for his services. Additionally, he kept our treatments simple and his wages modest.

If pharmaceuticals were necessary when I was a child, the doctor typically gave us some medication with our appointment so there weren't any prescriptions to fill. My mom usually didn't give us these pills. I never questioned her because she had healthy children that rarely missed school due to illness. Allow me to clarify; I missed school all of the time and my note always said the same thing: *Please excuse Christa, as she was ill.* But I was hardly ever ill. I just liked to hang out on the farm and do my own thing. Mornings were pretty hectic and it was imperative that we were self-starters. Initially, to save my mom time, I would write the body of my note for having missed school and have her sign it. To save her sanity, I learned how to sign her signature so she didn't know how much school I missed. I didn't want her to worry.

My career in wellness grew out of my passions from childhood. The path to my career, however, was not clear-cut. After leaving home for college, I began having debilitating migraines. Even though I was interested in natural medicine, I knew very little about it. Because I had moved away from my hometown, I was no longer seeing my family doctor and consequently began taking pharmaceuticals to manage the pain of my headaches.

My major changed many times because natural medicine wasn't an option and nothing else inspired me. During my college years, I longed for a career I felt was socially acceptable and financially promising. After completing 120 credit hours, I left with a gallimaufry of fading facts in my brain but no hope for a passionate career. While living in Boulder, I followed my true path and began my education in natural healing. In my late 20's, I co-founded the *Center for Wellness and Preventive Medicine* with a physician in Joplin, Missouri. I taught 8-week lifestyle modification workshops involving a vegetarian diet, yoga and meditation. At 31, I opened my own center without the medicine. Even though I was passionate about my vocation and continued to upgrade my health, I still suffered with severe headaches.

At 40, the frequency of my headaches increased due to the stress of divorce. My former husband and I parted ways as close friends but unpacking and putting away my dreams of having a family of my own was deeply upsetting. To help with the healing process, my best friend Lori encouraged me to spend a weekend with Tony Robbins. The event was radically transformational. On the first night, I walked barefoot on burning coals. The experience was liberating but the true gift was on the last day when he talked about nutrition. I had a long day of travel ahead of me and wanted to leave early because I didn't think there would be much for me to learn. I changed my flight and left. While I was in the airport, one of the friends I had made during the event sent me a text. Tony had challenged us to eat a 70% raw food diet for 10 days. My friend said,

"I committed you to the challenge by proxy." This altered the course of my life once again.

While researching raw foods, I found David Wolfe, a world-renowned educator on natural health and was inspired to commit to a nearly 100% raw food diet. I accepted Tony's ten-day challenge and raised him two additional years. During this time, I cleansed my body of the pharmaceuticals I had taken and removed toxins my body had accumulated from a mostly engineered food supply. My debilitating migraines ceased to occur and have never returned. Through the introduction of medicinal mushrooms, my immune system seemed invincible.

Being more connected to the environment on this diet, I replaced all of my cleaning and personal care products with environmentally friendly brands. Since my food was mainly raw, it was imperative that I not eat produce laden with pesticides or lacking in minerals. Therefore, the majority of my food choices were organic, homegrown or local. Frequently, I had superfood smoothies and fresh juices while increasing my intake of minerals and probiotics.

My water quality improved tremendously due to upgraded filtration and the addition of high quality salts. I reduced my exposure to EMF's, stopped watching television and spent more time outdoors. After reading the book *Food Not Lawns* (Flores, 2006), I turned the majority of my yard into a garden for growing food and medicinal plants. Infrared sauna sessions became a part of my weekly routine to improve the quality of my bloodstream. Tony had also encouraged us to rebound or participate in some form of fitness seven days a week. **My level of satisfaction and reverence for the world around me was directly proportional to my care of self.** Daily, I studied natural food nutrition becoming a BodyMind Nutritionist so that I could teach what I had learned.

FOREWORD

"People don't change"…"A leopard can't change its spots"… "You can't teach an old dog new tricks" – however you hear it, if you're stuck in your life right now, I *guarantee* there is some version of that playing in your head. And who could blame you? Living in a world with densely populated cities, filled with hundreds of sky-rise apartment buildings and businesses, it's easy to believe the world's problems are too vast to fix.

Yet what would happen if you could see the world differently – if the only thing that really had to change *was* your perception? What if you could see the world from a different view? What if your mind shifted and you no longer saw people with problems, but could see millions of people capable of making extraordinary and responsible decisions - including you - *especially you…?* Would it be a game changer for you?

It was for me. And Christa was my coach. Yet I resisted at first even though she'd been my friend for 30 years. I truly trust her with my life. But she wasn't the problem. I was. I didn't believe in me; I didn't believe I could actually DO it. So I told myself I couldn't.

If you're like me, you've heard it too many times to count: *All Change Starts with the Individual.* Gandhi delivered the message best when he said, "Be the change you wish to see in the world." And while I'm a great believer in this philosophy, I was always left wondering one simple thing…

How?

How can I change when no one else in my life wants to?

It was exhausting to be the spiritual black sheep in my family. At times, I felt like I was almost across the finish line to a new me when the old ways would draw close whispering, "If it ain't broke, don't fix it." Thus fueling the roller coaster ride of, "I think I can – Why bother – I think I can – Why bother – I think I can…"

In my 20's and 30's, I could ebb and flow with the direction of my life, healthy and happy. When times were good I'd coast. When they were bad I'd pray and gulp down new age thinking like a glass of delicious grape Kool-Aid after a hot day of handball. But when I hit my 40's my mind and body began to break down, refusing to bounce back like they used to. The high points felt insurmountable and the low points became my resting point.

And that's where Christa comes in. She's not a scientist nor would she want to be called an expert, even though many of her friends believe her to be one because she walks her talk. She's lived, endured and overcome every single challenge in her life by finding a way to be better off after each one. She doesn't focus on big changes as much as small shifts. Her goal isn't for you to change who you are - just how you think, with the grand outcome being incredible growth. You see, Christa expanded my mind, one tip at a time. And that's what makes her program special. It's why it's so *doable*.

Always a trailblazer when it comes to the connection between nutrition, mind, body and spirit, she's been known to take many an arrow from a naysayer. You might join that crowd after reading this book and say her ideas are unrealistic and resemble utopia. And if you do – I beg you – please read the book again.

Voltaire says, "Perfection is the enemy of good." Some feel if a plan doesn't solve every problem then good isn't good enough. This will only breed more excuses for you to stay the same. The point of *Mind Mirror* is to inspire you to move *towards* the direction of perfection rather than throw in the towel and give up hope that life can be better. And while this book isn't new age, I'd offer *isn't new age more fun to consider than old age?*

Here's the plain and simple truth: if Christa can do it, I know you can too. She actually lives the life she is teaching you in *Mind Mirror*. She did it with very little in terms of resources. Self-taught in many ways, her example will give hope to the millions of people who don't believe in their power to change their lives. This book is proof you can live a simple life and be truly happy without wealth, healthy without doctors and wise without having a Ph.D.

Mind Mirror was written as a part of Christa's crusade to spread the word of simplicity and sustainability. Her simple suggestions provide upgrades to your lifestyle so you can increase the power of your brain, improve your health and reduce damage to the environment. At the very least, it can point you in the direction of healing yourself and just maybe, heal our planet as a by-product of your process.

Let *Mind Mirror* serve as a reminder of the truth that is staring back at you every single day: in order to be happy, healthy and see the world transform, you just have to change yourself. As Christa will show you in this book, in order to be better at what you do, you have to practice; you have to keep learning. From practice comes the growth of new skills and ideas; Christa's unique perspective will restore hope in your heart for a happier life.

With uplifting encouragement she focuses on how you can "Be the Change" simply by shifting your perspective towards sustainability and ultimate health. And while *Mind Mirror* may not go so far as to reinvent the wheel of a natural lifestyle, if you're feeling a little stuck in the mud like I was, I guarantee Christa can get your wheels turning again. With a few simple steps, you'll be well on your way to discovering a better version of you.

Join her on her journey to leave the world in a better place than she found it. And just maybe your grandchildren won't have to be filled with wonder about the wilderness, the same way we were about space at their age. And just maybe, if we all do a little better we can leave a legacy of pollution free air, clean streams and an earth filled with natural resources to sustain love, life and liberty.

Lori R. Taylor

ACKNOWLEDGMENTS

I could have written a book about all of the positive impacts the people in my life have made. Each member of my family has contributed to love and understanding bringing me peace each day. My friends and clients have brought so much laughter and wisdom that I can't thank them enough. As for the countless people in my life who have helped me to learn the *hard way*, I offer my sincere gratitude.

Special thanks to Lori Taylor, Teena Franklin, Ree Wells, Jay Engelbrecht, Bruce Jones, Ann McGregor and Nate Williams for encouraging me to refine my message. Your suggestions and edits were very much appreciated.

It was the best of times, it was the worst of times,
it was the age of wisdom, it was the age of foolishness,..
Charles Dickens *A Tale of Two Cities*

Even though we may at times feel powerless to change the world, we should never quit striving to be better... for the children.

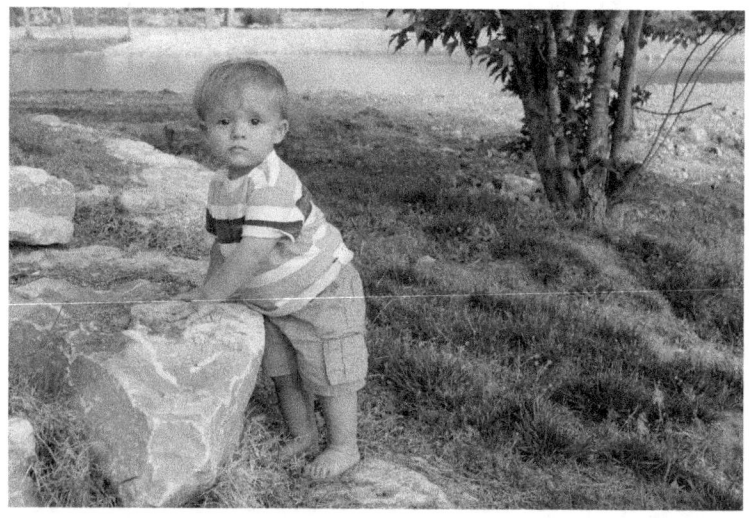

Unless someone like you cares a whole awful lot,
nothing is going to get better. It's not.
Dr. Seuss

INTRODUCTION

We have a wealth of knowledge at our fingertips about how to heal our lives. Even with the best of intentions, relationships will end, our nutrition will suffer and times will change without warning. Life presents us with many difficulties. It takes courage to approach it with an open heart and hope allows us to feel that one day, we will be more satisfied. However, due to increasing toxicity in our mental and physical environments, people are starting to doubt that *this too shall pass.* Many struggle with the consequences of a stressful lifestyle and need a paradigm shift. Due to poor lifestyle choices, we're not fully activating our genetic code. By living holistically, we can reach deeper levels of consciousness. Nutrition affects mood and our relationships. By upgrading our lifestyles, we can improve our mental and physical health. When we're experiencing peace in our bodies and minds, we can set more noble goals and transform our world.

Unfortunately, many people are becoming more immune to the destruction of the planet and less immune to the destruction of themselves. At times, my viewpoint clouds my ability to fully enjoy the world around me. According to my mom, I have a charmed life and need to be grateful instead of dissatisfied. It's difficult for her to understand my quandary about the human experience but I firmly believe we are capable of being so much more than we actualize. I tried to explain to her what I meant by asking, "What if your grandchildren came home from Disney Land and you told them they had to sit in the living room and watch the Disney Channel? They would soon tell you they were bored and mean it with all of their hearts. They've just been thrilled and astonished and now you expect them to sit inside your house, watch television and *Love* it?" She replied, "If they complained after having been taken to Disney Land, I would tell them they're spoiled."

I guess I'm spoiled then because I want to be thrilled and astonished, everyday. However, my dream is to be amazed by activating more of my DNA - not a Disney gift card. If it's true that we have vast amounts of untapped brain function, I want to tap it. While studying nutrition, I learned about the function of our cells. They are filled with thousands of protein machines that need minerals to function. The word "protein" comes from the Greek word *prota*, meaning *of primary importance*. Knowing that our food supply is nearly devoid of adequate minerals, leads me to believe my cells are filled with potential energy that is waiting for me to access it. Many of our cells don't receive the proper care to survive, let alone thrive. By improving the function of our brain cells, we can improve the function of our brains. As we activate more of our genetic potential, I feel our opportunities to be thrilled and astonished will increase exponentially.

Sadly, the forced march to acquire possessions, make lots of money and be accepted in a capricious society consumes most of the energy needed to satisfy the basic requirements of our brains. Enzymes also contribute to the functioning of our cells and they begin to decline in our 30's. The toxicity of our environment contributes to the destruction of our cells, as well as the delicate organisms that call our bodies home, sending us on a slippery slope as we age. The statement that youth is wasted on the young is apropos. For when you finally realize what you want to do with your life, a fair portion of what you may need biologically is already gone.

In our current society, many people are in stress. A large portion of this stress is due to inadequate nutrition. Deficiencies in necessary minerals contribute to stress in the body, which leads to stress in the brain. When the brain is in stress, your perspective towards life is affected. By operating mostly from one part of your brain over another, you influence how you see the world. When feeling peaceful, you activate the healing and repair systems in the brain. When your body and mind are in states of harmony, higher consciousness is possible. If you're in physical or mental stress, you activate the regions of your brain responsible for fight, flight and freeze. This response is related to survival and it disrupts true creativity and peace of mind.

For many years, we've heard that changing our thoughts alters our brains. Sometimes it's difficult to change your thoughts because of a lifetime of false beliefs about yourself. However, in many cases, a lack of love or poor nutrition is causing us to experience stress in our brains, affecting the way we view the world.

Part I of *Mind Mirror* begins with my journey on the road to health. Part II includes ideas and resources for reducing stress in your body to shift your brain into the frontal regions responsible for inspiration and transcendence. For when we access higher states of mind, we might see how our current way of life was possibly created because we were stressed and by shifting our perspective, we might truly change the world. My hope is that one day society will head towards more sustainable, peaceful ways. Turning this complex system around will be similar to making a U-turn with a train, so I don't anticipate it will be immediate. I do feel we need to reduce our speed towards destruction. At the very least, we need to look at where we're headed with hopes that the light at the end of the tunnel isn't another train.

PART I

HIGHWAY TO HEALTH

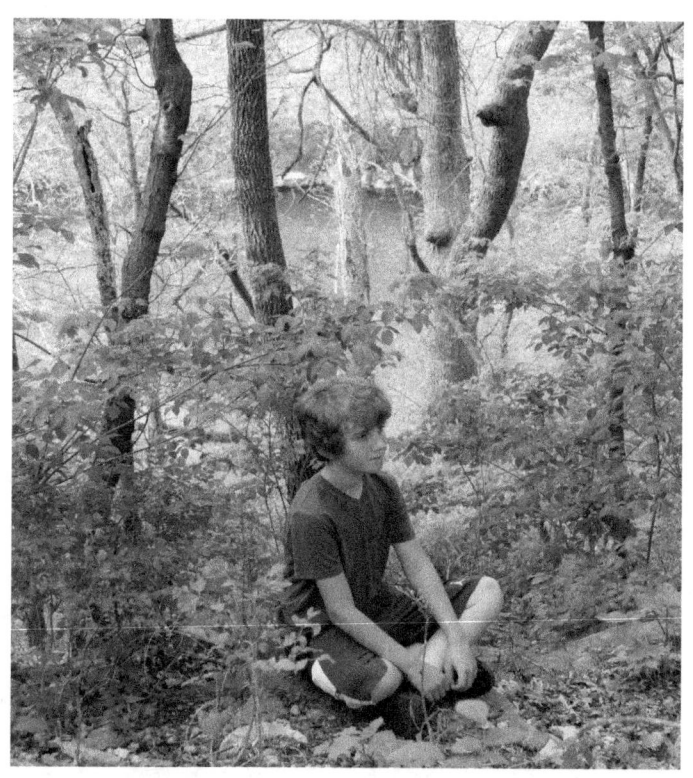

Humankind has not woven the Web of Life;
We are but one thread within it.
Whatever we do to the web, we do to ourselves
All things are bound together;
All things connect.

Chief Seattle

CHAPTER 1

TO THINE OWN SELF BE TRUE

I think the reward for conformity is that
everyone likes you except yourself.
Rita Mae Brown

Traveling on a high-speed train in China, my brain could not process the staggering number of factories, dormitories and trash heaps along the coastline. It might feel good to buy something beautiful from the opulent department store but if you had to go in the back door of one of these factories to do your shopping, it would curb the appeal. The unintended consequences of materialism were vivid. Clearly, the air quality was polluted so the food and water couldn't have escaped contamination. I began to wonder, *how are my actions contributing to the destruction of humanity and the environment?*

A few days into the trip, I visited an embroidery museum where photographs were not permitted. During the tour, I was told about this art form that takes decades to master. There were only 12 masters of this style in all of China. The guide led me to a woman using a needle and thread on fine silk and said, "We've had her since she was five." She was an apprentice and wouldn't reach mastery for possibly decades. I couldn't gauge her age, maybe 25 but her eyes looked sad and the thought that they *had* her like she was something you could own was unsettling. Possibly his choice of words misrepresented her participation at the museum, but nonetheless, I was visibly disturbed. I gave her a compassionate smile; she never spoke. He led me into a separate room to view the masterpieces. Words will not describe the beauty of these exquisitely embroidered silks, some selling for over a million dollars. The thought of the girl's servitude, the dedication of one's entire life to the true mastery of a skill and seeing such magnificence all at once brought on a deluge of emotion. Until that moment, I had never been moved to tears by art but the tears they came as he gave me the history of each piece. I was hoping he wouldn't ask me about my physical reaction because I certainly couldn't explain. Throughout the tour, the tears continued to come and my heart grew heavy. I left the museum and tried to shake the somber mood but it was no use.

> *In the middle of the road of my life,*
> *I awoke in a dark wood to find the true way, wholly lost.*
> Dante

Being in China was a living metaphor for my life. My world was upside down, night was day, and due to the time difference, it was both yesterday and today at the same time. I was leading a double life. In the months leading up to my visit to China, two of my best friends had died of sudden illnesses, my grandmother had passed and my former husband, whom I cared for deeply, had died tragically in a plane crash. Significant people whom I turned to for inspiration and identity were gone. My trip to China was intended to reconnect me with my spirit and peace of mind. For 15 years, I had been in the field of wellness and natural food nutrition. Through cleansing and a purified natural diet, I had cured myself of migraine headaches and improved my weakened immune system. However, in the weeks following the deaths of my loved ones, I had taken departure from my healthy lifestyle. My purified way of life had separated me from most people. Longing for connection instead of isolation, I strayed from nature and my spirit slipped away from me into the dark wood.

Due to stress in my body and mind, I was not activating the regions of my brain responsible for happiness and, consequently, I felt a lack of hope for transforming myself or my community through nutrition. When I looked around, instead of seeing promise, I saw people suffering even though they were trying to live healthier lives. With all of our potential, people were still struggling to find peace, to heal, to create a better world for future generations. With all of our progress and understanding, we continued to drive the world on a crash course. I began to think it was too late to heal the world. Certainly, I was starting to doubt *my* ability to make a difference.

The Chinese New Year was approaching and the train stations were filled with people leaving their factory lives, returning to their villages. This mass exodus for many marks the only time of year they will see their families. This realization was sad enough; seeing them loaded down with the very materialistic goods they've sacrificed their lives to make was disheartening. Often you hear if you stop buying from China it will help remedy the problems with the factories. Sadly, they were contributing to their own demise. Some people say if they didn't have these factory jobs, they would die of starvation. This thought was even more disturbing since the next city I arrived in was among the wealthiest cities in China. Upon arriving there and seeing vast fortunes, I had an epiphany. The Chinese need to take care of China; I'm going to focus my attention on myself and my local community.

> *Here is a test to find whether your mission on*
> *earth is finished: If you're alive, it isn't.*
> Richard Bach *Illusions*

After returning home, I had a very difficult time feeling peace. I knew the changes I needed to make in my lifestyle would lead me back to separation and consistently being faced with defending my way of life and my philosophies. No one else in my circle was fully committed to my lifestyle, so I would have to toe the line alone. Most people don't want to be reminded of the sadness that lies behind consumerism and factory farm food. I had enjoyed *belonging* again but I also knew deep down inside that it would ultimately be unsatisfying if I weren't contributing my efforts to the greater good. Even though I had tremendous resources to reclaim my spirit, it continued to slip away from me.

I recalled the girl in the museum and wondered, what would I want to master if I was going to devote my life to something? The only answer that came to mind was *my mind,* namely, due to the fact that I wasn't feeling peace. Being alone was a constant reminder of the deaths of my loved ones. I had not fully processed their absence. Regularly, I tried to meditate but I couldn't shift my consciousness back to the lively place it had been prior to losing them. Feeling a lack of energy, my enthusiasm for nutrition was low. All of the methods that had once connected me to spirit were not working. Even while in nature, I did not hear the voice of the earth.

Attempting to keep my mind on the present moment seemed futile because the moments felt bleak. Eventually, I realized my perspective of suffering was due to a combination of physical and mental disharmony. Having strayed from my purified lifestyle, my body was in subtle stress and I was functioning from the survival regions of my brain instead of the areas responsible for higher consciousness. In order for my meditations to be truly effective, I would need to cleanse my recent transgressions.

Having studied various educators on natural nutrition, I expanded my horizons beyond a raw food diet. Diligently, I improved my nutrition and attempted to meditate daily. I considered how much easier this would all be if I were in love but I was not involved and was in no position to pursue a relationship. During this time, I wished that feeling self-love was as magical as feeling love for or from another. Then I began to wonder, could it be possible to actually *feel* self-love with the same amount of emotion? By tuning my mind and body towards self-love, would it simply alter my attitude or would there be a physiological, palpable change? If love truly comes from within, then maybe it wasn't someone else's love I had felt in the past, maybe it was something that came from me. Possibly, it was a feeling I had tapped into because my mind was intensely focused on love. Periodically, I tried to meditate on self-love but continued to feel disconnected. Having returned to a purified diet, taking medication or drinking alcohol was not an option to reduce the pain. As difficult as this time in my life was, I knew if I did not fully address the underlying causes, I would never truly experience peace in my body or mind.

One night I awoke at 3 a.m. in a troubled state. Intensely, I focused on my breath with my attention centered on my heart. Finally, I felt relaxed enough to fall back to sleep with a quiet mind. When I awoke, I could feel the shift. Having fallen asleep in this state, I must have entered a deep place of healing. Without any outside influences coming to rescue me, I was at peace and felt like I was in love. The feeling I was experiencing was an all enduring, unbreakable, perfect love from within. It was similar to the kind of feeling I have felt being fully present in an awe-inspiring place in nature. Only this time, *I* was the beautiful place in nature. I did not need affection from another to feel this love; I was the source and the recipient. The spell of heartache and loss had been broken.

Over the next few moments, I made many realizations. I recalled things I had done and remembered places I had escaped to, in order to remedy pain. What I needed had been with me all along. It was like a road map of my life laid out and the words "You Are Here" spelled out in my mind. Consequently, the words "and you were here and here and here" followed. I had missed many opportunities for healing because of this one lesson: **Love comes from within.** Realizing that I had not been in tune with self-love, to this degree, was fairly profound information.

Even though one might be able to survive without love, I concluded, without *feeling* self-love, one wouldn't reach self-mastery. I realized that I needed to be focused on the breath to feel self-love. They seemed to be linked and in that moment, they became one and the same for me.

Breath + Love = Self-Love

It's easy to get pulled into the drama of life and lose connection with spirit and lose awareness of yourself. Therefore, mindfulness is absolutely necessary to stay aligned with this feeling. Maintaining an awareness of the breath and love throughout each and every day is absolutely necessary for making lasting change. It may not feel profound to read these words but the practice of regularly meditating on self-love was deeply transformational. For me, it became easier with practice. All I would have to do is breathe deeply and a chill would rise up my spine. I would instantly feel centered and aligned with my higher self. I still become overwhelmed at times over the loss of my loved ones but by breathing deeply and focusing on self-love, I'm able to feel connected to them and to myself. Now I feel certain, the love that never leaves you, regardless of circumstance, is self-love.

Empty calories, drugs and alcohol lost their appeal when my life was focused on self-love and the goal of reaching my genetic potential. In order to activate more of my DNA, respond to life with ease and continue to improve my brain function as I aged, I knew I needed to continue to upgrade my water, my food and get more oxygen to every cell in my body. In order to prioritize these requirements, I asked myself, how long could I live without food, water, air? The actual numbers varied but on average I knew I could live about three minutes without air, three days without water and three weeks without food. These were my basic needs for survival and each day should be prioritized in order of their importance. If I wanted to thrive, love would need to be woven into the tapestry as well. These prerequisites for self-mastery were so intertwined I could not think deeply about one without touching on the other. Often times, I blend these subjects because I believe we are love; we are mostly composed of water; we are what we eat.

I found it interesting to look up *composition of the human body* in Wikipedia. The article claimed humans are 57% water. The mass of water is majority oxygen even though more atoms are hydrogen. Therefore, by mass, we're mostly made of oxygen. We breathe to take in oxygen and I like to believe the breath is love. Therefore, in my view, the air we breathe and human body is mostly composed of love. When I read the entire composition of the body, it was easy to see the old adage *you are what you eat* is generally true or as Michael Pollan, author of *Omnivore's Dilemma*, puts it, "You are what you eat eats."

The breath was my number one priority; I didn't want to take it for granted. When I was stressed, my breathing was shallow and less oxygen was delivered to my cells. Making the effort to breathe deeply throughout the day assisted me in attaining a proper mixture of oxygen and blood, improving the function of my body and mind. Being mindful of the breath while feeling love was even better. My goal was to maintain awareness of higher consciousness, cultivating a mind and body that supported me in reaching my genetic potential.

DAILY PRIORITIES :
Number 1: Breath (Love) + Number 2: Quality Water +
Number 3: Quality Food ⇨ SELF-MASTERY

CHAPTER 2

AMERICAN EVOLUTION

We do not inherit the earth from our ancestors;
we borrow it from our children.
Chief Seattle

One evening, an elderly Cherokee brave told his grandson about a battle that goes on inside people. He said, "My son, the battle is between two wolves inside us all. One is evil. It is anger, envy, jealousy, sorrow, regret, greed, arrogance, self-pity, guilt, resentment, inferiority, lies, false pride, superiority and ego.
The other wolf is good. It is joy, peace, love, hope, serenity, humility, kindness, benevolence, empathy, generosity, truth, compassion and faith."
The grandson thought about it for a minute and then asked his grandfather, "Which wolf wins?" The old Cherokee simply replied, "The one that you feed."

While on the path to recover my spirit, realizations about why people are not reaching their potential became clear. When our bodies and minds are in stress, we cannot clearly see the trap that binds us. When the body is in stress, the brain is operating in a mode of survival. Without being connected to the regions of the brain responsible for higher cognitive function, most solutions will be based on fear. In order to access these regions of the brain consistently, physical and mental needs will need to be met, regularly. In order to experience vitality, one needs to emotionally, physically and mentally, detoxify the body.

When I used to teach classes on nutrition, I would suggest people make small changes and slowly incorporate healthier choices. However, throughout my adult life, I've settled for small improvements and minor setbacks for so long that it felt like I was going sideways. When I fully committed to a holistic lifestyle and raised my level of responsibility for the environment, I experienced profound benefits. I've felt heightened intuition and creativity. My thirst for knowledge has been insatiable so every day I try to learn something new. While I'm getting ready for work or preparing food, I'll watch an educational video or listen to a podcast. It feels good to be in a state of growth and I love to share what I've learned.

Being in the field of wellness, I've met amazing people working to transcend the concerns of our complicated world. I'm sure it comes as no surprise however, that the majority of people find their way to my center for two reasons, weight loss and stress. Over the years, I've heard of many nutritional plans but their downfall, in my opinion, is a matter of semantics. The word "diet" comes from the Greek word *diatia*, meaning *way of life*. If the word diet essentially means weight loss for you, then your way of life must support this goal. The failure happens when you realize that a way of life based on a singular objective is destined for failure. For if your entire way of life does not support your goal, how can you succeed? A way of life should honor all of life. Since most people have lives that reach far beyond the bathroom scales, one must look at the issue from another angle. How is my way of life contributing to my weight? The answer may seem obvious but the question that follows may not be so clear. How does my way of life respect all of life?

My struggle has not been with weight; it has been with stress. When I took the time to see how my way of life respected all of life, I saw many factors that contributed to my stress. I began by noting how

I actually spent my time and money. My actions were not always supporting the macrocosm of Earth that supported life. Nor were they supporting the microcosm of cells and beneficial bacteria within my body. I was not eating to support the health of the microcosm. My monetary choices were not supporting the wellbeing of the macrocosm. When I began to live a way of life that supported both, my results far exceeded my expectations. Maintaining my ideal weight was a natural consequence of my lifestyle, not the objective. Having a way of life that supported all of life fostered a happier life for myself and a better world. The unintended benefit of this shift was the cessation of my headaches.

Expanding my awareness to the environmental consequences of my choices supported a life of reduced stress. This more responsible way of life gave me additional motivation other than health risks for improving my nutritional decisions. I became more aware of how my choices were affecting the environment and by reducing toxicity of the earth; I concurrently reduced my exposure to toxins. By examining the ingredients of the cleaning products in my home and business, I found most of these ingredients were harmful. Our bodies will produce fat to store toxic substances if they are not excreted. Sometimes exposure results in rapid onset of illness but usually effects such as a weakened immune system and hormone dysfunction are less obvious. In general, as my level of conscientiousness increased, the respect for my body increased and I began to honor myself more. Raising my awareness of the environment improved my self-reliance and provided greater peace of mind.

Taking away the symptoms of stress did not solve my problems. Reducing my stress in the middle of a battle was never possible. Preventing the battle was the best course of action. Creating a lifestyle based on peace and harmony within my environment was ideal.

Initially, I didn't realize how big of a role my brain played in this process. I knew I needed it to survive but by not making continuous effort to keep my brain out of stress, all of my goals became harder to attain. It was helpful to know that my brain consumed a tremendous amount of energy. My body and brain were competing for the food I'd consumed and if I wasn't conscientious with my nutrition, both my body and my mind suffered. If my brain was not getting what it needed, my perspective shifted to survival mode. When this happened, I was hindered at learning, I was not able to feel true peace or potential and it affected my mood, which affected my relationships.

In addition to being mindful of the brain, I had to reduce my scope to the microcosm of delicate cells and mircoflora inside my body. We have trillions of beneficial bacteria in our bodies and these benevolent little creatures work laboriously to help us digest our food and contribute to the functioning of our immune systems. By maintaining a large population of beneficial bacteria in my body, harmful bacteria would not overpopulate, potentially causing an illness. If harmful bacteria were treated with antibiotics, beneficial bacteria would be eliminated as well and my immune system would continue to struggle. As I reflected on the consequences of medications and alcohol, I realized the effect these substances would have on these tiny cells and beneficial bacteria. If drugs can kill a human, certainly they can kill cells and beneficial bacterial. When deciding what course of action to take to heal, I considered the community inside my body. This holistic view raised my level of care and personal responsibility.

Being aware of the far-reaching consequences of my choices, made me vigilant about caring for myself physically and mentally. When I was experiencing stress, my view of the world was very narrow and usually self-serving. By thoroughly meeting my needs, my vision

12

expanded to consider humanity and the brain that connected us all, the Earth. The environment was a big concern; therefore, I made an effort to reduce my ecological footprint. Unfortunately, I didn't realize all of the little things I was doing each day that contributed to further contamination of the planet. To improve my role, I examined every dollar I was spending. By having greater knowledge of the companies that lacked environmental responsibility, I could make more informed decisions about where to spend my money. To my misfortune, the majority of the grocery store shelves are filled with products made by companies that fail when it comes to environmental responsibility. Due to this fact, it has taken more effort to raise my level of care but I've made many positive discoveries in the process. Fortunately, there was a book and an app for my mobile phone that rated companies based on quality, reliability and scope, as well as social, political and environmental factors.[1]

The book and the app both contained numerous categories to assist me in upgrading the quality of my purchases, making my actions more responsible. The *Better World Shopper* application for my mobile device was convenient when in the store. By improving the quality of my purchases, I improved the condition of the world. The problems we face politically, socially and environmentally are immense; many claim they are too widespread to change. Fortunately, I felt I was making a difference with every dollar I spent when I stopped supporting companies that further contributed to the issues that threatened a more conscientious way of life.

The Better World Shopping Guide paperback assisted me in making more informed decisions. The first book I bought is now outdated because the author, Ellis Jones, Ph.D., consistently gave companies opportunities to improve their score. Unfortunately, some changes were due to smaller, once reputable companies being bought by less responsible companies trying to capitalize on the healthy brand name while lowering all of the standards they once upheld. Now, I prefer to use the app that is constantly updated and more convenient.

Many people ask why I want to take in all of the negative information about corporations but I firmly believe knowledge is power. I am inspired by data that helps me take the best care of my body, my mind and the environment. In todays' world we're bombarded with pollution, chemicals, electromagnetic fields and an alarming array of degenerating factors. It's in our best interest to improve our choices to the highest degree in order to be healthy. Consuming pure water and food helped cleanse my body and improving my sources for information assisted with cleansing my mind. When I raised my level of awareness to include the world around me, I began to set more responsible goals and experienced more rewarding relationships.

During the years I was creating my garden, I was able to see a very close connection to the soil and the immune system. Healthy soil is teeming with organisms all performing necessary functions to maintain the ecosystem. We have a similar eco-immune system inside our bodies. Without healthy soil, I would not have truly healthy plants. Without healthy food or a healthy inner ecosystem, I would not have a truly healthy body. When I'm ill, my body goes into battle for survival. I am essentially at war with myself.

In 1918, Randolph Bourne stated, "War is the Health of the State." The health of a nation can be determined based on whether or not it is engaged in war. Battles are rarely contained, whether they are in a country or an individual. Prevention of disease is the best cure for the body; this theory holds true for a country as well. The best way to improve the health of a nation is to improve the responsibility of its people. Unfortunately, many people in this country are physically and mentally in stress. Over the last 100 years, with all of our amazing discoveries, why have we not found lasting peace?

Looking back over my own life, I realized energy that could have been used to make a positive difference in the world was being devoted to appeasing societal whims. Being concerned with the bigger problems facing the world barely made it onto the radar when I was battling the signals from my own body and mind. To our misfortune, people experiencing stress run the world. If our leaders don't take the time to restore peace in their bodies, how can we ever expect them to have a vision of true peace in their minds? As long as the people of a nation continue to function in survival mode, we will continue to elect leaders based on fear instead of peace.

Embracing a more natural lifestyle, I cultivated a deeper connection with the planet. Being more in tune with the earth enabled me to make more connections to the world. Everything is connected. For me, humans represented the microcosmic forces of the macrocosm. Connections between the soil and the human body were found. The interrelation of my body and mind became more apparent. Parallels were drawn between the war in my body and the war amongst countries. Similarly, a lack of personal responsibility was mirrored in the land, the human body, our health care system and government.

When insects are found on plants, many people spray pesticides to exterminate them. When harmful bacteria are found in the body, antibiotics are prescribed to destroy them. When infection is recurrent in the tonsils, recommendations are made to remove them. When people in a foreign country are disruptive, plans are made to attack them.

Instead of so much killing and destruction, we should find out why plants and the human body are too weak to fight off disease. It's wiser to find out why people have tonsils and address the reasons for their recurrent infection. We should respect human life and not kill innocent men, women and children in the wars we send young adults to fight.

It came as no surprise that there was so much dis-ease in the world. The human body is not given a fair chance to reach its genetic potential because people are gambling with poor water and inferior food. We are increasingly becoming less self-reliant for our survival or as Daniel Vitalis, a leading health and personal development strategist, put it, *surthrival*. In today's world, food, water and virtually every creature comfort must be provided. Being disconnected from a truly independent lifestyle leads to increasing dependence.

Most people are working the majority of their lives in hopes one day they can retire with enough energy and money to enjoy their freedom. My dream is that soon, we will all be living more simple lives in tune with nature, in the prime of our lives. I envision us enjoying peace of mind and reaching our ultimate potential, instead of being enslaved to a system of poor health and consumerism.

By understanding biological processes and becoming aware of the consequences of my actions, I experienced a shift in values. If society shifted, we could work together to heal our land. For in order to reach self-mastery and truly honor our existence, we must honor the land that makes our lives possible. My prior way of living was unsustainable, even if it brought me happiness at times. When I took the time to listen to my inner voice, I heard that I was not as happy as I wanted to be. Until I made radical change, I didn't truly feel how much potential I had. If we collectively activate more of our genetic code through enlightened nutrition and self-love, we could transform our world and hopefully reduce suffering.

We don't need a revolution in the United States.
...What we need now is an American Evolution.
Swami Beyondadanda

PART II

STAIRWAY TO HAVING

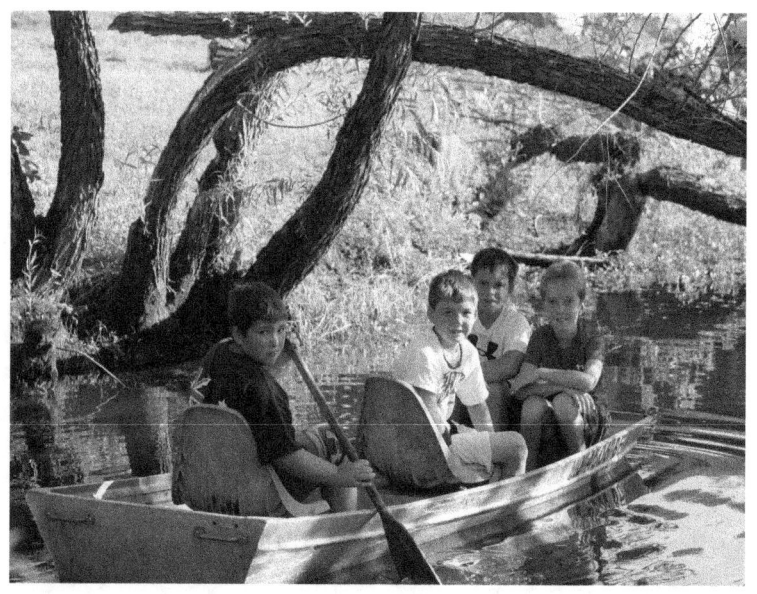

There is a magnet in your heart that will attract true friends. That magnet is unselfishness, thinking of others first; when you learn to live for others, they will live for you

Paramahansa Yogananda

CHAPTER 3

BE-LOVE IN YOURSELF

Re-examine all you have been told..
Dismiss whatever insults your own Soul.
Walt Whitman

Be the change you wish to see in the world. This saying by Gandhi represents personal responsibility. If you are upset about the state of the world, you need to first change yourself in accordance with your ideals and values. These days, it seems the change we need most in this world is to feel we are truly loved. Since all change starts with the individual, it's important to begin with loving yourself.

There is a story of Nasrudin, the wise fool of Sufi folklore, who was in the courtyard looking in the dirt. A bystander asked what he had lost. Nasrudin replied he had lost his key. The man joined in the search and after some time, he asked Nasrudin, "Are you sure you dropped your key out here?" Nasrudin replied, "No, I dropped it inside but it's dark in there and I can't see."

It's overwhelming to process the lengths we go to feel love when we're out of tune with self-love. Whether we acquire material possessions, over-consume food or move from one relationship to the next, we try to feel love outside of ourselves. Many people have the wisdom to recognize they are searching outside of themselves for love but still we look in the courtyard. The key to feeling love is within but the darkness of rejection, loneliness and confusion makes it very difficult to spend too much time looking inside ourselves. In the dark, we draw the conclusion we are to blame for lacking love. Even if you feel you did nothing wrong, rejection will take its emotional toll. If we rely on another to make us feel loved, we have not only lost our key, we don't believe it belongs to us in the first place. In *The Path to Love* (Chopra, 1998), Deepak tells us; eventually we will adjust to the darkness and be able to see more clearly. Rumi asks, "And you? When will you begin that long journey into yourself?"

There are countless books on love and loving ourselves but we often hear these words in our minds with little change in our hearts. Occasionally, bits and pieces of truth make their way into our awareness but the meteors of our perceived reality crash into us throwing us off course time and time again. The idea of self-love has always been there but the notion of tuning to it has been given little attention. It's as if self-love exists on a specific frequency and it's necessary to align with it. Take a moment to consider the following questions. Are you comfortable with yourself when you are alone? If you lost everything you own and everyone close to you, would you feel whole, complete, loved?

The worst loneliness is to not be comfortable with yourself.
Mark Twain

We tell ourselves, as long as we are loved, we'll be fine. Yet even with love abound, we feel a deep loneliness at times. The hardest thing to accept is you may have abandoned yourself, albeit, unknowingly. Most people don't realize they're out of tune with loving themselves because someone or something is always filling the void.

We believe that loving another person is all we need in order to feel love. Many times I've heard the saying: "You cannot love another until you love yourself." When you feel you're a loving person it's easy to conclude that you must love yourself. However, why do we feel unloved when a relationship ends?

Can you tell a difference between love that comes from yourself or the love you feel from others? Is it even possible to feel love from another person or does it all come from within? The answers are difficult to discern. Consider the possibility that when you miss another person's love, it's not them you miss but how you've felt about yourself when you were with them. If it all comes from within, you can recreate loving feelings without them. Potentially, throughout our lives, we've been out of tune with this awareness because we've attributed our feelings of love and magic to someone or something outside of ourselves. It's a little easier to distinguish self-love from love you receive from others when you're experiencing the loss of a relationship. When you feel the heartache of a breakup or a fight with a loved one, can you sit quietly with yourself and feel a perfect love? You may not but it's in these moments that you'll need self-love the most.

A common thread in my life has been an awareness of the present moment or meditation. Focusing within the moment allowed me to have reverence for my surroundings and a peaceful quiet mind. However, realizing that I had not meditated on self-love provided light in the darkness. It was the key I had been missing. Spiritual teachings tell us you don't need any special skills or accomplishments to feel love. Love truly comes from within; it is everlasting. It cannot be damaged or wrong. It cannot be taken away or lost. You don't have to believe in it but I have come to discover, you do have to breathe in it.

Attuning to self-love takes a concentrated effort. For the next few moments, close your eyes and tune into your breath. Without attaching any thoughts to your feelings, allow an awareness of self-love to fill your being. Depending on your current circumstances, this may be a difficult meditation exercise. I encourage you to sit with this feeling repeatedly throughout the day. Self-love is a divine reality words fail to describe. It's a state of being with which you consciously have to align yourself. Like a pilot always correcting his course, you must adjust your awareness to a state of self-love. If it's challenging for you, know that it will get easier. With practice, eventually, you'll be able to tune to feelings of self-love in an instant. When you're truly in touch with this feeling, physiological change will occur. If it doesn't, keep working on it. Similar to when you think of someone you're in love with, sensations will be palpable.

Feeling self-love can be difficult, especially if you are in pain. With sudden and traumatic injuries, our bodies have systems that seal pain from our awareness for survival. Unfortunately, for many people, pain is chronic, not acute. For years, I have suggested *mindfulness* to deal with chronic pain. Often people find it's the inner voice surrounding the pain making it intolerable. Our thoughts about the limitations of pain or possibly the financial costs of pain are compounding the problem. Awareness and a quiet, peaceful mind can reduce symptoms immediately.

Pain is often emotional not physical, therefore, a lot of this information is directed at emotional stress or *perceived* reality. When it comes to emotional pain, the part of your mind that suffers is the part you've constructed to protect yourself during times of struggle. It takes time to create this system of protection and it will most likely take time to dismantle it. Reducing physical or emotional pain may require a rewiring of your mental construct. This will involve a diligent effort to release pent up emotions and quiet the constant companion in your mind, the inner voice. We would like to believe this voice is reasonable but if we were able to record it and listen to it throughout the day, we would find it is often mistaken, quite insecure and incessant. It is difficult to actively listen to the voice and maintain a state of true calm and awareness. Cultivating a quiet mind that observes without judgment is best.

I remember reading once about the difference between believing and knowing. Believing meant you didn't know. The question was put to me like this: If you were standing with your back to a clock and someone asked you what time it was, without turning to look, would you know the time? Based on various details you may *believe* you know the time but without actually seeing the clock, you wouldn't *know* for sure. The voice inside is the *believer*; the loving observer of your reality is the *knower*.

In *The Voice of Knowledge,* Don Miguel Ruiz describes how we came to trust our inner voice and why it's often misinformed. Our minds are filled with misperceived stories about ourselves and the people in our lives. Ruiz tells us, "Just because you hear a voice in your head it doesn't mean that it's speaking the truth."[1] Since childhood, we've been trying to please others. In many cases, we're looking for acceptance from people who are not in tune with their mental, physical or spiritual potential.

Our brains will construct many realities for us. Some of these constructs are based on instinct, some are based on consciously processed information and some have to do with the ability to seam the two hemispheres of the brain together. When the corpus callosum, a membrane allowing the two sides of the brain to communicate, is severed, the right doesn't know what the left side is doing.

Michael Gazzaniga, a preeminent brain scientist, observed fascinating behaviors while studying split-brain subjects. In one study the word *walk* was presented to only the right side of the patient's brain and instantly the subject got up and started walking. The interesting part is when the question about why the patient was walking was presented to the left side of the subject's brain (the part that didn't hear the word *walk*) he gave a reason for his behavior, without hesitation. In this case, the patient claimed he wanted to get something to drink and he *believed* that is why he was walking. [2]

The experiment demonstrated how quickly a person would suggest a rationalization for something he doesn't truly understand. The two sides were unable to communicate but the desire to justify behavior was rapid and seemingly unconscious. There are many implications to this information. Even though these findings are based in a malfunctioning brain, they provide clues to the rapid ways the mind will attempt to make sense out of reality it doesn't understand. It's a rather fallible system, but the need for survival has taught us to hone the skill of making quick assessments.

The next time someone does or says something that triggers an unpleasant reaction in you, pause. Take a moment to consider that even though you have come up with a reason to justify your reaction, it may not be the real reason you were activated. Breathe deeply, center yourself and see if possibly your way of life was challenged, causing you to shift into survival mode.

In the book *Blink: The Power of Thinking without Thinking*, Malcolm Gladwell explains how unconscious behavior can shape our actions. We make split second decisions we're not fully aware of in order to size up our surroundings.[3] When I took the tests available online to demonstrate the role my subconscious played in my decisions, I was shocked at the results. Even being aware of the programmed biases I was experiencing, I still had difficulty making "quick" decisions based on my "conscious" choices because the tests were too rapid for processing. My choices were subconscious and I had to repeat the tests with sharper awareness to sway the results. Search for IAT tests by Gladwell to experience examples of your unconscious behavior.

In the book *The Power of I Am,* John Maxwell Taylor teaches that eye contact can affect the way people receive you. He explains that looking into a person's right eye with your right eye, may trigger their personality (ego) but looking into their left eye with your left eye acknowledges spirit and indicates a desire to make a meaningful connection with another. This all depends on whether or not you are right or left-handed. Your personality eye is the same as your dominant hand.[4]

After reading this material, I immediately used the technique in a store. Just by having the intention of making a meaningful connection with another, created a heightened state of awareness, even if I was the only one to fully realize what was happening. I do notice a difference in how people react to me when I approach my interactions conscientiously. This is a win win technique.

We must remind ourselves daily that people are struggling with problems of their own. By allowing trivial matters to steal our energy we're taking time away from feeling love and connection with others. Understanding all of the ways our minds prevent us from feeling peace will help remove some of the anxiety and fear. If we raise our level of interacting with everyone we come into contact with, we will transform our lives. Consider the fact that you most likely don't have enough information to judge anyone, especially yourself. In order to stay connected to the positive flow of progress, we need to make a conscious effort to move past difficult feelings as quickly as possible.

I used to have a cat. Sometimes she would come up to me wanting affection but if I was distracted for whatever reason, I might not engage in giving her attention. Every time I was aware enough to catch it, she would walk away and immediately shake her body. It was as if she wanted to discharge her feelings of rejection. It's a good practice to let go of negative energy soon after a stressful event if you can. Just having the intention to release negative energy helps the situation. Raising my level of interaction, even if it's only with myself, makes a difference.

How many times have you allowed emotions and self-doubt to lead your mind into a state of fear or stress only to realize later you were completely wrong? If you had plans with a friend and they didn't call, you might create all kinds of reasons out of insecurity and fear. Later, when you've found out they tried to contact you but your phone wasn't working, all of the fears are lifted. These episodes of misguided responses are rampant. However, for many of them we don't get the opportunity to discover the real truth. If we knew the amount of misinformation we had received, we would be stunned. If we were able to dismantle self-limiting beliefs created out of misinformation, we would be liberated. With this in mind, why would you want to give absolute authority to the often erroneous inner voice or believe in criticism from another?

In *Notes to Myself,* Hugh Prather says, "A criticism is at best a description of the immediate past. It does not describe the future course of a life."[5] Your opinion of me is a reflection of you, not of me. Additionally, it describes the past and says nothing of who I will become in the future. Letting go of hurt feelings is difficult but it's much easier if you do it immediately following the infraction. It's much harder to let go of energy you've stored and possibly solidified in your body.

When I lived in Boulder, I studied an energy bodywork technique called Polarity Therapy. I know it sounds a little *out there* but the things I felt were absolutely *in here*. By in here, I mean, I felt movement from another body inside my own. The process involved putting my hands on someone and feeling the gentle rhythm of their energy. The best way to get you to feel what I'm talking about is to rub your hands vigorously together, close your eyes, be very still and stop rubbing your hands as you barely separate them. You will feel a wave-like motion or pulsation and attraction of energy between your hands. With practice, you can put your hands on someone and feel this subtle ebb and flow in their body. The purpose was to get blocked energy moving, to assist in healing.

There were many experiences worth noting but one has stayed forefront in my memory. On one occasion, I had my hands on a woman and could feel the rhythm. Then she remembered something from her past she wanted to share with me. It was a painful memory and as soon as she started to tell me about her experience the flow stopped and all I could feel was tension. The change was similar to a subtle vibration verses a wavelike motion. I asked her if she could stop telling the story for a moment and take deep breaths until I could feel the wave again. Once the feeling resumed in my hands, I encouraged her to proceed slowly with awareness of the breath and this time she was able to get a little further without the tension but soon it was there again. We repeated the process, stopping the story and resuming deep breathing, every time I felt the tension. It took her entire session to tell me a story she could usually tell in a few minutes. However, taking the time to let go of the charged emotion surrounding this pain was worth the effort. In the end, she admitted the story no longer activated her the way it had in the past and hopefully, she no longer feels that painful memory. Imagine how much easier it would be to let go of difficult emotions if you rapidly restored harmony in your body instead of hanging on to pain as a way of protection.

Looking back, I can recall times I've hung on to negative feelings towards another. I'm not proud to admit that occasionally I was trying to teach someone a lesson. For if I immediately forgave their indiscretion, then they essentially *got away* with something. I felt that if I let their bad behavior slide time and time again then I would see more bad behavior. It's taken a while to realize this reaction is very ineffective.

You may never be able to influence or modify another person's behavior. The only person you have the power to control is yourself. Usually, there is so much more information about why a person acts poorly than meets the eye and reacting to limited information, will produce limited benefits. Additionally, you are the one who has to feel the negative emotions you cling to, regardless of the reason you cling. Practice Nonviolent Communication (NVC) to raise your level of awareness and improve your interactions with others.

To be effective in releasing negative feelings, it's important to occasionally tune out your inner voice. During meditation you will find the inner voice is POWERFUL. It will take more than a few moments of concentration to keep it at bay. It will take diligence. Life is busy; we don't all live in monasteries where we can sit in meditation all day. It's best to practice awareness of the present moment regardless of your activity. Attempt to expand your attention to your hands and feet at the same time you're reading this book. It's ideal to listen to others while simultaneously maintaining an awareness of your body. This helps keep your mind focused and your perception centered in the present.

Surely, you've experienced your mind wandering while driving. After a certain amount of time, you have to ask yourself, *how did I get here?* It was the constant observer that allowed you to lose focus without an immediate accident. However, the observer is at the mercy of your attention. At some point you'll have to reenter this space to control the circumstances before you. When your mind is centered in your body, you will move and respond to life with more efficiency. Evenly dividing your awareness between your body and mind will prevent you from becoming lost in thought and reduce the occurrences of physical injury. With this technique, you'll have a calmer, less emotional awareness of your surroundings. The inner voice can't command your total presence if your body is holding some of your attention.

For the next few moments, bring your awareness to your right foot. If it's safe for you to do so, send all of your attention there. Notice the intricate details and sensations. Can you stay entirely focused on your foot while simultaneously thinking about a nice memory from childhood? Are you able to recreate all of the specifics and emotions from your childhood memory while feeling the subtle sensations of your foot? I've found it's impossible to place 100% of my attention on my body and maintain any clarity of thought and vice versa.

During the next emotional storm expand your awareness to your arms and legs. You can center yourself by feeling the expansion and contraction of the breath. Remember the surface of the water can be rough but there is calm in the depths. When you reach these calm states, fill yourself with the feeling of love. Once you've slowed your pulse rate, meditate on your heart center. You are more than a body. You are more than a mind. Your grounded, quiet presence gives blessings to both. Practice body-centered awareness and restore harmony by tuning to self-love.

It may take effort. Love is like a garden. Gardens need to be tended with trust that the plants are growing beneath the soil. You can't dig up your carrots daily to see if they're maturing. You can't plant a seed and walk away, especially in the beginning stages. Nurture a tender awareness to fully establish your love of self. You can't just read the words. You will have to feel them deep inside your being. Once you do this, you'll no longer need to believe it, you'll know it.

It's subtle, but the problem with self-love arises when people don't recognize they're not loving themselves. Saying *I love myself* is like *saying* the word food instead of *eating* food. Food only makes you full when you consume it. The key is, you have to *feel love* just as you have to actually *eat* food to experience satiety. You could begin by saying *I love myself* then after a few repetitions remove the word *myself*. Breathe this in while repeating *I love*, then remove the *I*. When you feel love, maintain a silent presence of this awareness and smile. If you don't feel truly loved regardless of circumstance in your life, keep focusing on it. Keep searching inside for the keys to unlock your heart. True self-love is there waiting for you.

Each day needs to be prioritized according to what you need to thrive. Most importantly you need to breathe. First thing in the morning, upon waking, you should sit quietly with your breath. Be mindful of the notion that your breath is your body's way of expressing its love for you. They say you can't go three minutes without the breath and I would like to take it deeper and say you shouldn't go three minutes without truly loving yourself. As many times a day as you can, breathe in the feeling of self-love.

Maintaining a state of loving awareness will be more effective than periodic reflection during times of trouble. You can't eat healthy for a day and expect to maintain good health for a lifetime. In the same respect, you can't feel self-love once and expect to sail through life, happily ever after. Let go of negative emotions soon after you feel them. With a heightened state of awareness and the intention of making meaningful connections with others, the occurrence of negative experiences will hopefully diminish. Realize that many of the people causing you pain are in pain themselves. Most of this pain is based on misinformation so have compassion when true understanding isn't an option. Be gentle with yourself and others. Forgive. Effort must be maintained to thoroughly and radically transform your life but you won't regret it. When you take time to *be-love*, everything changes.

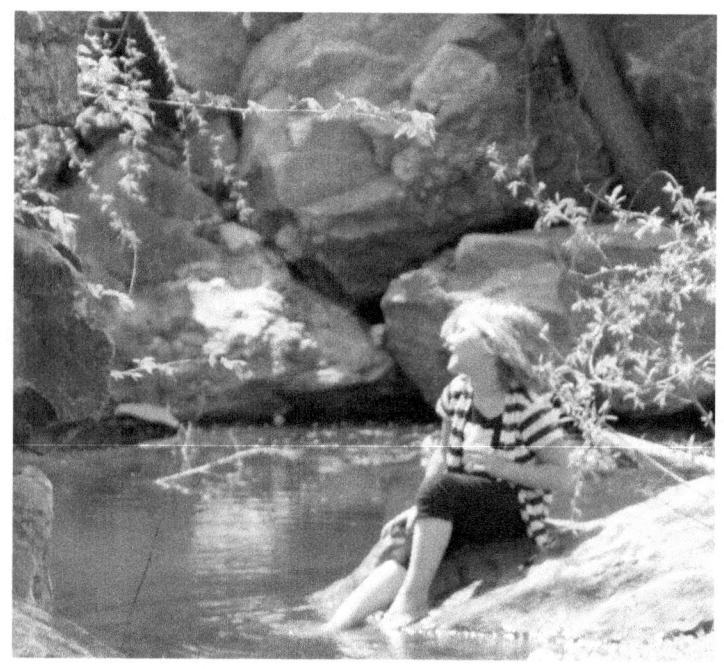

Now I see the secret of making the best person: it is to grow in the open air and to eat and sleep with the earth.

Walt Whitman

CHAPTER 4

MESSAGE IN A BOTTLE

In the world there is nothing more
submissive and weak than water.
Yet for attacking that which is hard and
strong nothing can surpass it.
Lao Tzu

Staying connected to spirit is easier when you're respecting and loving your physical form. You will not survive without water and you cannot live a masterful life without quality water. The first lesson I learned in my nutrition education is there are always upgrades. It may seem like a lot of effort to research and learn new ways of being healthy but remember, you're an extraordinary being and you should make extraordinary effort to care for yourself. I'm very passionate about nutrition so I spend a tremendous amount of time learning about the benefits of proper sustenance. The most intriguing thing I learned in my studies is that ionic trace minerals lower the surface tension of the cell. This means drinking water with these minerals actually allows more water into the cell providing for better hydration. These minerals are also necessary for cell function. Without adequate minerals, the cell will not reach its genetic potential. The cell may survive but it will not thrive. Imagine how different you might feel if all of your cells began to function at a higher level?

Considering your basic needs, the priority following the breath is water. In the morning, water will assist your body with waking. You've been fasting all night long and now it's time to break the fast with breakfast. Before you have coffee or a meal, Lars Gustafsson founder of The BodyMind Institute, suggests a morning drink. Add a 1/2 a cup of organic juice to a glass of pure water, 5-10 drops of ConcenTrace® Trace Minerals and a pinch of high quality salt. I'll give more details about the benefits of this drink in Chapter 6.

We've been taught salt is bad for us and for the most part, this is true. The minerals in processed table salt have been destroyed and this form of salt contributes to many adverse health effects. On the contrary, high quality salts such as Antarctic, Himalayan and Celtic sea salt are instrumental in restoring cell function. The 84 trace minerals found in high quality salt are necessary for the activation of enzymatic reactions in our bodies. Every system and organ in your body needs minerals to function. We have a lack of minerals in our food supply; therefore, the addition of high quality salt in our water will activate more of our genetic potential. David Wolfe recommends sea salt above rock salt.[1] It's strongly recommended that you know the source of your supplements. I've listed trusted suppliers for salt in Appendix II.

> *All of us have in our veins the exact same percentage of*
> *salt in our blood that exists in the ocean, and, therefore,*
> *we have salt in our blood, in our sweat, in our tears.*
> *We are tied to the ocean.*
> John F. Kennedy

Avoid bottled water that comes in plastic. I'm sure by now, it's common knowledge there is an area twice the size of Texas in the ocean littered with plastic. Another reason to avoid plastic bottles is they off-gas for a year and need to sit before being filled. However, most plastic bottle manufacturers immediately fill their bottles once they are blown. Additionally, elements in plastic are leached from the bottle into the water.[2] Your body will use what you give it if you don't give it what it needs. It would be beneficial for you and the environment to carry your water in pure stainless steel canisters, glass or at the very least, in eco-friendly reusable water bottles. I prefer to wash and reuse glass jars.

I'm not a fan of most popular commercial mineral waters because I've learned the minerals need to be ionic, in order to lower the surface tension of the cell. The accumulation of minerals that are not readily utilized in our bodies can contribute to stone formation and arthritis. Not all mineral waters are created equally. In order to make a more informed choice, start by looking up your favorite brand of water in the *Better World Shopping Guide*. You might be surprised to find your company of choice gets an F. F companies are actively engaged in some of the worst environmental and social practices in their industries. Furthermore, the claimed health benefits of F companies may be exaggerated or blatantly false. Instead of wasting money on bottled water, I filter my water with a Berkey filter and fill reusable glass bottles for transport. The Berkey filter is gravity fed, meaning it will filter your water in the event of a power outage. A set of Berkey filters will purify 6000 gallons of water and the purification elements are self-sterilizing.[3]

If you don't filter your water before you put it in your body, your body will become the filter. Our systems are already so taxed; this small effort will make a big difference. Placing trace minerals back into the water returns it to a living state. Living beings experience greater harmony by consuming living water and food. Having access to pure spring water would be ideal but unfortunately, this isn't an option for the majority of the population. Therefore, improving the quality of water available to you is necessary for true health.

Don't assume your unfiltered tap water is healthy to drink. Medications and environmental pollutants can end up in the water supply. Additionally, chlorine damages the delicate micro flora necessary for digestion and immune function. Fluoride interferes with magnesium delivery and impedes pituitary function. It contributes to acidic states in the body, affects digestion and disrupts thyroid and hormone function.[4] I'm not declaring whether or not fluoride is harmful for your teeth. I'm merely suggesting our ability to thrive is hindered by its addition to our drinking water. The Center for Disease Control has expressed that the allowed amount needs to be lowered to protect the public's health.[5]

If you have concerns with your well water, a solution would be to distill the water then add quality minerals. If you have city water that isn't filtered my suggestion is to purchase a Berkey or Pro-Pur filter. Filter your water and store it in 2.5-gallon glass jugs. This size will be easier to handle, especially if you are using them in a water dispenser. After filtering the water, always add minerals. Use a pinch of high quality salt and 5-10 drops of trace minerals for every liter of water. Adding high quality salts will improve cell function but they won't be able to efficiently run systems like digestion, detoxification and nutrient absorption, especially if these systems are not fully functional. The ConcenTrace® drops will further assist with these systems.

Drink water throughout the day but if possible, avoid drinking during meals. Beverages, including water, will hinder digestion. For some, it is socially fun to drink wine or other beverages with meals but this will affect digestion. Occasionally drinking with meals will be okay but if this is a regular habit, you should work on modifying it. A simple rule for calculating the amount of water to consume is to take your body weight, divide it in half and drink this amount in ounces. Of course if you are out in the sun, exercising or using saunas, you should increase the amount of water you drink. Sweat comes from the movement of water from the blood plasma. Using a far infrared sauna is an excellent way to detoxify the body and blood stream. Replacing lost fluids after an infrared sauna session with high quality water and trace minerals is an ideal way to improve the quality of the blood.

Hormone function is improved by consuming purified, re-mineralized water. Lars Gustafsson teaches that all hormone function is electrical.[6] This electricity is supplied by electrolytes. Electrolytes are vital for communication across the cell membranes and for emitting impulses to other cells. This communication is especially important for your nerves, heart and muscle tissues. You can make your own high quality electrolyte drink with purified water, ionic trace minerals and a splash of organic juice. Sweeten it with raw honey or agave if necessary. Skip the high sugar sport drinks with dyes and inferior water, sold in off-gassing plastic bottles.

What could you do to improve the environment? Most everything you pour down the drain, ends up in our rivers and aquifers. Remember what you don't filter out of your food and water, your body must filter for you. In the same respect, the municipalities must filter harsh chemicals you allow back into the water supply. Just as your tax-dollars subsidize the production of the highly destructive corn syrup industry, your hard earned wages are paying for the purification of your drinking water. Based on the products you use in your home, what could you change to improve the quality of the water? Go through your cleaning supplies then look up the company you use in the *Better World Shopper*. Keep in mind that vinegar is a perfect cleaning solution for almost any household surface.

Most people reply on water from their faucets verses learning ways to naturally collect water. With a gravity-fed water filter system and rain barrels you could have clean water, especially in times of emergency. Filter your bath and shower water to remove chlorine at the very least. Chlorine damages the beneficial bacteria on your skin and breathing chlorine gas is harmful to your health. The skin is the largest organ in the body and it will absorb impurities.

Clean water is necessary for cleansing and restoring vitality. When it comes to vibrant health you will also need a clear conscience. Dr. Masaru Emoto claims that thoughts can affect the structure of a water molecule. In his book, *The Hidden Messages in Water*, he states, "What we imagine in our minds becomes our world."[7] His experiments on water molecules have led some to believe the water in our bodies is affected by our thoughts. In the same regard, one might conclude clean water contributes to a clear mind.

Possibly you've heard the phrase; *water seeks its own level*. It raises the question, if I'm mostly composed of water, then at what level do I exist if my water is contaminated? Mark Sircus, Ac., OMD, states, "The costs of distancing ourselves from the purity of consciousness and the purity of water are astronomical." The second most important aspect of your survival is water. Are you giving this life force the respect it deserves? Approximately 70% of the earth's surface is covered in water. Clearly, we need to raise our level of awareness to honor its role in our existence.

CHAPTER 5

THRIVING BIOLOGICAL ECONOMY

For all the environmental troubles single-use shopping bags cause,
the much greater impacts are in what they contain.
Susan Freinkel

You will live roughly three weeks without food, but if you want to improve brain function and unlock more of your genetic potential, you're going to need access to healthy food. It may be helpful to think of your food choices like a monetary system. Unfortunately, most people are nutritionally in debt but with a few upgrades you can restore balance. When it comes to the body, it craves minerals but our food supply is starkly deficient due to commercially grown food from big agriculture monopolies. Poor food choices are similar to bad investments.

Charlotte Gerson from the Gerson Institute explains that commercial factory farms don't start with adequate minerals.[1] Of the 52 elements needed, the average commercially grown plant starts with about three. The health of the plant is dependent on these 52 minerals. Without them, the plant is susceptible to pestilence. These conditions are combated with pesticides, herbicides, and fungicides, not to mention genetic modification. Fruits and vegetables reach the peak of their nutritional value in the last few hours of ripening. However, commercially grown produce is picked several days before ripening. Once it's picked, it will no longer receive nutrients from the earth. As a matter of fact, the nutrients will start to decline once the fruit or vegetable is disconnected from the mother plant. During the days to follow, harvested produce will lose approximately 50% of the nutrients it once had unless it's been carefully stored in a root cellar. The average piece of produce will travel 1500 miles to the local grocery. Distribution centers artificially ripen some produce by exposure to ethylene gas before delivery to the store. No one knows how long it was separated from the earth before it reached your dinner table. You can know it was never allowed to reach its genetic potential from the initial planting and it will have declined rapidly in value by the time you consume it. This plan will not provide a healthy return for your investment.

In learning to care for an organic garden, I became very familiar with all of the nutrients it took to make the soil healthy. When I realized the harm being caused to the environment by supporting monoculture, I could not eat factory farm food in good conscience. The unfairness of government subsidies, genetic modification, herbicides, pesticides and fungicides further motivated me to reduce the intake of mega farm food.

You will survive on what you are given but you will not thrive if you are given substandard, counterfeit food. Through biological transmutation, dangerous metals will be delivered to your bones and tissues when the necessary minerals are deficient. Your body will attempt to convert cupcakes into calcium but this doesn't take place in a vacuum. There will be consequences to improper nutrition. Ayn Rand once said, "You can ignore reality but you can't ignore the consequences of ignoring reality." Rand is a controversial individual but when you apply this quote to the treatment of our bodies, it's difficult to dispute. Are we taking extraordinary care of our bodies, minds and the earth? Foster Gamble, in the documentary *Thrive*, asks, "Is this really the best we can do?"[2]

It goes without saying the majority of the population has a poor nutritional foundation. The Standard American Diet fittingly has the acronym, SAD. Too many people are not reaching their potential when it comes to love either. This is sad on a more intrinsic level. We crave love when we're not loving ourselves. Your body has a similar reaction to food. If your body is craving minerals for biological function and you deprive it of these minerals, it will crave more food. You'll never have a feeling of true satiety until you feed your body the correct minerals. You may fill your body with an over abundance of the wrong food and fool your body into feeling its needs have been met. Yet in times of dis-ease, your body will no longer be fooled by the inadequacies of your choices.

If you were to feed your body impeccable nutrition, you may or may not experience dis-ease but you'll have considerable more control over your fate should you be subjected to a physical ailment. Most likely, you won't find yourself in the hands of a doctor for primary care if you're primarily caring for yourself. Your body can divinely guide itself through the healing process. Similarly, the health of your love-life won't be at the mercy of a lover if you feed yourself an abundance of positive beliefs and allow yourself to feel self-love, at all times.

In order to have a thriving biological economy, I would suggest eating as close to nature as possible. Due to an inadequate food supply, supplements are most likely necessary. Do your research and find whole food verses synthetic supplements. Try to find out how these supplements function in your body. What systems do they affect and how did those systems become dysfunctional? Taking the latest supplement to be promoted on television without having a holistic view of your body is not recommended.

When it comes to the human body, you should familiarize yourself with these processes: Digestion, Absorption, Utilization and eXcretion (DAUX).[3] If you don't have nutrient delivery or waste removal systems in order, then supplementation may not be beneficial. There needs to be a holistic view of the body when supplementing, not a singular objective, like losing weight. Additionally, medications can alter absorption and metabolism of nutrients. Food can affect absorption, metabolism and excretion of medications. Some medications and supplements could be thought of as loans. They can get you by for a while but if you want to be solvent, you'll need to repair the problems, not quantitatively ease the pain or mask the symptoms.

Chemically laden, genetically modified food is similar to borrowing from a loan shark. The interest is painfully high. Drinking pop is like doing business with gangsters. This habit will do physical and environmental harm. Your body will need about 32 glasses of water to neutralize the effects of one can of soda. Environmentally, the BPA from the cans, water pollution from processing and litter from the plastic is not worth the supposed satisfaction.[4]

Cleansing is similar to paying off your debt. People often talk of cleansing without making permanent changes in their lifestyle. They detox so they can *retox*. The average person has 2-20 pounds of toxins stored in their gut, fatty tissues and cells. However, doing a cleanse before your DAUX systems are online is like using your Visa to pay off your MasterCard. It will ultimately be futile, especially if you don't commit to a purified lifestyle. Know that it takes less energy to maintain a healthy body than it does to repeatedly restore it.

Are you consuming a currency your body can't spend? Are you accumulating a debt your body is struggling to repay? The time is right to invest in high quality food. There is a wealth of knowledge to be gained from nature. To secure a sustainable future, it would be wise to keep your interests local and reduce the outsourcing of your health.

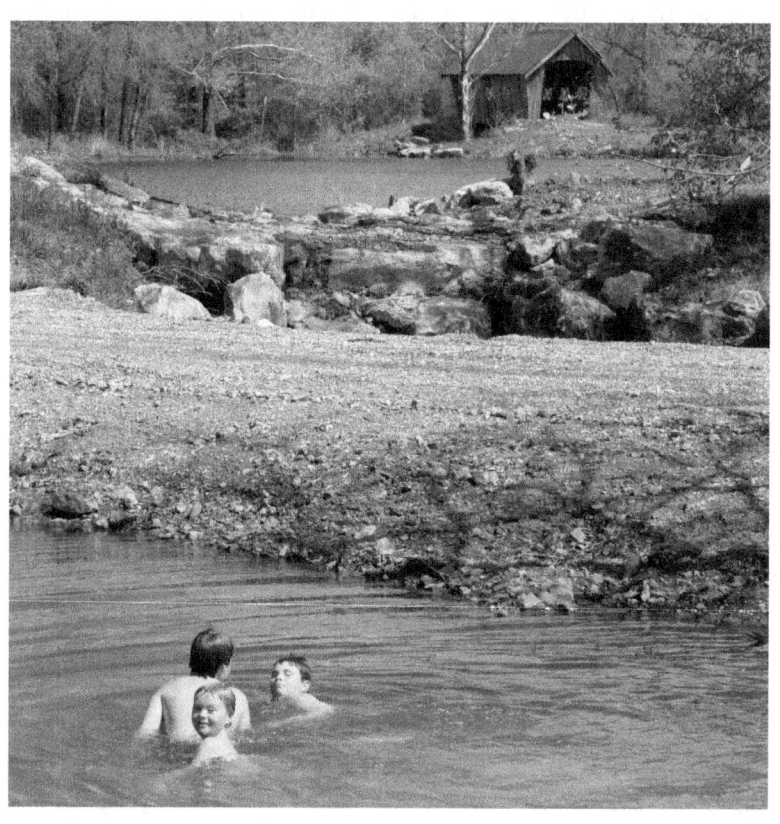

There is new life in the soil for every man. There is healing in the trees for tired minds and for our overburdened spirits, there is strength in the hills, if only we will lift up our eyes. Remember that nature is your great restorer.

Calvin Coolidge

CHAPTER 6

BODY LANGUAGE

In the 21st century our tastes buds, our brain chemistry,
our biochemistry, our hormones and our kitchens
have been hijacked by the food industry.
Mark Hyman, M.D.

Honoring the vast connections within your body and nature will contribute to true health and happiness. In Lewis Thomas' essays *The Lives of a Cell*, he discusses the connection between nature and humanity and how imperative it is we understand the role we play in this relationship. He sheds light on the fact that we do not fully understand Earth yet we have the technology to destroy it.[1] The same is true for our bodies. Thomas is not a pilot but claimed he would rather be given the controls of a 747, than to be responsible for the functioning of his liver. He stated, "If I were informed tomorrow that I was in direct communication with my liver, and could take over now, I would become deeply depressed."[2]

This statement puts into perspective the intricacies of the human body and how fortunate we are that mostly it can function without our conscious control. However, in order for your body to be effectively self-regulating, you need to give it proper care. Your body is the most magnificent thing you will ever be given the power to influence. In order to produce the food intended for us to consume, we will need to improve our relationship with the planet.

According to Wikipedia: *"The Golden Age* denotes a period of primordial peace, harmony, stability and prosperity. During this age, peace and harmony prevailed; humans did not have to work to feed themselves, for the earth provided food in abundance. They lived to a very old age with a youthful appearance, eventually dying peacefully, with spirits living on as guardians."

My hope is that if we reach mastery of our bodymind processes and live in harmony on Earth, we can return to the *Golden Age.* Improving our relationship with ourselves will be instrumental in this process. Everyone knows in order to foster respect you have to listen. The language of your body becomes quite clear when you commit to understanding. In order to open the lines of communication, you'll need to tune into your hormones. The hormone system is a complex communication system. Hormones affect all processes in the body, as well as your mind. You can begin to restore balance to this system by adding ionic trace minerals found in high quality salt. Think of these minerals or *electrolytes* as a secretary in an office. If she isn't fully present and prepared to do her job, she will miss incoming calls, transfer calls to the wrong offices or take down incorrect messages. This will create stress in the malfunctioning office, affecting all relationships in the work environment.

The hormones can be thought of as the key players in the workforce. In this scenario, everyone is highly and specifically trained to do their jobs. However, if key players aren't getting their messages, this will cause even more malfunction. Sometimes, other players will pick up the slack but if this kind of thing continues over time, these players will get burned out on their job and not function very efficiently. As with any system that is designed to function in a specific way, it will not run optimally if there is long term inefficiency. This labor force may be very forgiving but it may not forget. It certainly won't appreciate being ignored or taken for granted. Key players (hormones) may decide to strike or quit all together. You could think of organs as departments in an office. If things get bad enough, the boss may decide that a whole department (organ) needs to be removed. Unfortunately, the system will suffer greatly if this department isn't replaced. Depending on what was substituted as a replacement, the potential for more dysfunction is possible.

When you stop taking responsibility for your body as a whole, there will be trouble. It may go unnoticed at first but continued abuse will affect your ability to sustain a truly healthy body. When you decide that your gal bladder is no longer necessary and you have it removed, you will miss it. I'll say it again, nothing happens in a vacuum. Take a moment to look up the reason why you have a gal bladder; it isn't an accident. I know there are many scenarios I can't comprehend where surgery is the only option to improve quality of life. However, many people opt for a radical surgery when radically improving their lifestyles would correct the problem. To me, the latter isn't actually radical. If missing a meal causes your brain stress, how do you think it feels about missing an organ?

Understanding hormone function is vital to your health. Insulin is a key player in the hormone system. Some refer to it as the master hormone and resistance to this master will create a cascade of problems in the body. If you are insulin resistant verses insulin sensitive, your cells will not be fully functional. Most people who are not diabetic are not particularly concerned with their blood sugar but they should be. Not managing your blood sugar properly can cause your body to be in a state of stress all day long. It contributes to reduced metabolism, fat storage, lowered digestion, blood pressure issues, insulin resistance, and a lack of oxygen to the cells. There are many consequences to ignoring the sensitivity of this system and unfortunately everything from electromagnetic fields to artificial sweeteners will play a role in how it functions. Repeatedly going too long without a meal or consuming too much sugar in one sitting will set off a chain reaction in your body resulting in higher levels of cortisol (stress hormone) and reduced peace of mind.

Low, steady insulin levels will have a very positive effect in your body. Dopamine levels are affected by insulin. Lower than optimal dopamine levels are linked with insulin resistance. Consequently, this combination is connected with addiction and pleasure seeking behavior since dopamine is related to reward and pleasure. In essence, meal timing and higher quality food can lessen addictive behaviors. When you are sensitive to insulin, proteins (chains of amino acids) are more fully utilized in your cells. Each cell is a little protein factory. By balancing your blood sugar throughout the day, the more efficiently your trillions of factories will perform. Much of the protein we consume is not utilized and if your processes of elimination are not functioning properly, the waste material will become impacted in your intestines. With proper protein function, you could improve your ability to release toxins and body fat while increasing muscle tone.

Think of impaction as the home of a hoarder. The hallways are so filled that you can't reach your destination. In this analogy, nutrients can't get effectively delivered and waste can't get adequately removed. It takes about one minute for blood to circulate throughout your body. If you are not eliminating waste or toxins, this matter is recirculating throughout your bloodstream and being deposited into bodily tissues. Imagine a polluted river overflowing the banks depositing waste around your city 1000 times a day. The stress of this contamination alone creates more work and tension for our bodies. We lose vast amounts of energy trying to utilize the improper food we consume. We produce fat to store the waste we can't excrete. It would be so much more efficient to improve the systems in our bodies and spend less money on food and supplementation. We would also spend less money on medicine as well. All the while we would have more energy to love and fully enjoy our lives.

To simplify the subject of proteins, enzymes and amino acids, think of them as building materials. Some of these materials we create and some we need to acquire. The more efficiently we create and assemble building materials inside of our bodies, the fewer materials we need to consume. Overeating is a sign of inefficient systems. Don't settle for this malfunction. Regardless of your story, upgrades are available.

Optimizing cell function, combining the right foods and properly timing your meals can improve the insulin system. Managing blood sugar is paramount to health and it can be greatly improved with a few adjustments to your lifestyle. A BodyMind Nutritionist can provide individualized recommendations with regards to managing blood sugar and overall nutrition. Consider watching the film, *Simply Raw: Reversing Diabetes in 30 days*.[3] Research the work done by Gabriel Cousens if you are struggling with insulin health related problems. Your doctor should closely monitor any recommendations made in this book if you are diabetic.

If your body is telling you it's time to eat then most likely you've already waited too long or possibly the quality of food you've chosen has deprived your cells of what they truly need. The hunger signals are your body's way of asking for a remedy. Your brain isn't getting what it needs and the stress response to follow will prevent you from seeing the world in its entire splendor. By developing a deeper understanding of your body's language, you will reduce stress in the body. When balance is achieved, the survival responses deployed by the brain, can retreat. After harmony is restored, peace and greater vision is possible. With equanimity in your body and mind, your reactions to life will be more conscientious.

When life is approached with a calm presence, decisions will be made that reach beyond a limited worldview. With a holistic approach to caring for your body, you will feel more complete, have more control over your life and experience greater power. When our responses to life are less reactionary, more responsible solutions can be generated. Voltaire said it best when he said, "With great power comes great responsibility." A holistic lifestyle requires effort but the returns are immense. For a moment consider the possibility that all of the problems in the world were created because the people making decisions are physically and mentally in stress. As a people, if we reduced stress, preempted problems and reached harmony within ourselves, maybe this wave of peace could reach beyond our bodies into our world.

CHAPTER 7

SEE JANE THRIVE

*The art of medicine consists of amusing the
patient while nature cures the disease.*
Voltaire

The body is an interconnected system that doesn't thrive with a truncated viewpoint. When you approach life holistically, you start to see the body is like an elaborate spider web. You cannot touch a strand without the entire web feeling the effect. M. Scott Peck begins *The Road Less Traveled* with the sentence, "Life is difficult."[1] However, improving food choices and nutrient delivery systems will ease a life of strain. The first thing you can do to reduce stress is to breathe. Five deep breaths are enough to lower cortisol levels and shift your brain into a more peaceful state. Take deep breaths prior to a meal to aid in digestion. In addition to aiding in digestion, deep breathing will activate your parasympathetic nervous system, improve immunity, as well as insulin sensitivity and hormone function. The parasympathetic nervous system is associated with states of healing and repair.

Digestion is regularly overlooked when it comes to a healthy body and mind. If you're not properly digesting your food, you're in essence wasting the money you spend on food. Would you be happy receiving only 50% of your pay each week? By not making the effort to keep your body out of stress, you utilize, on average, 50% less of your nutrients. This alone causes the body even more stress. The first phase of digestion begins in your mouth. The simple process of chewing your food will greatly improve digestion. During your next meal, count the number of times you chew your food before swallowing. Most people only chew their food 5-15 times. Make an effort to chew each bite at least 20 times. Smoothies and blended foods are a great way to assist the breakdown of nutrients. Having superfood smoothies like the ones recommended by David Wolfe will give you an amazing boost to your health. Additionally, blended foods will be a blessing for those struggling with the inability to effectively chew their food.

Hydrochloric acid (HCL) is necessary for digestion. Unfortunately, due to stress this substance is decreased in the stomach. Stress creates acidity and affects the pH level of the blood. In order to regulate pH one of the places your body will seek neutralizing agents is from the salt in the HCL. Many people who suffer from heartburn believe they need to take antacids. When stomach acid drops *too low*, the sphincter at the top of the stomach will fail to close. This results in a backup of stomach acid into the esophagus, causing pain.[2] Taking raw apple cider vinegar or hydrochloric acid pills containing betaine can assist in raising stomach acid and preventing heart burn. Antacids will mask the symptoms but they won't address the underlying problem, therefore, this cycle will continue until you care for the cause. Drinking mineral water with your meals will interfere with HCL. It is predicted that about 50% of the population has lower than optimal HCL.

Another supplement you could add to your diet to improve digestion and cell function is digestive enzymes. Metabolic enzymes are found in every living cell. They are biologically active proteins.

Enzymes (chains of proteins) run the cell. All metabolism is enzyme based. Therefore, enzymes directly affect metabolism. The number of enzymes you have or produce reduces with age. Stress, calorie restriction, toxicity and cooked foods all contribute to the depletion of enzymes. Enzyme depletion contributes to the aging process. Raw foods contain natural enzymes to assist digestion and cell function. Most traditional cooking methods destroy the enzymes present in food. If you are predominately eating cooked food, you should consume supplemental enzymes. Because of deficient enzyme processes, we are not fully activating our genetic systems.

Consuming a majority of raw foods in your diet will assist with the maintenance of your health, as well as physical and emotional cleansing. Most raw-foodists are very focused on the quality of food they're consuming. To the best of their ability they eat organic or local food if they're not growing their own. Being concerned with where your food is coming from brings you closer to the actual environment. Growing your own food establishes a direct relationship with the earth. When this relationship is cultivated, you become more aware of the condition of the planet. By raising your consciousness, you actively participate in recycling, composting and using eco-friendly products.

Previously, I touched on the acid/alkaline system in the body. It's a very complex system but I'll simplify part of the process. The pH of your blood will need to be maintained at approximately 7.36. If your body becomes too acidic it will leach calcium and other minerals from areas such as your bones, muscles, teeth and tissues, as well as the aforementioned HCL to help alkalinize the body. Stress in the body causes acidity. The more acidic your body is, the greater decrease of enzyme and DNA function, as well as lower water cell volume. Many foods have an acidic reaction in the body. There are several websites that provide acid/alkaline food lists. It would be helpful to view and print one of these lists.

Dairy is very acidic so I've never understood the "Got Milk" ads. Well, I understand they're deceptive. They suggest the calcium in milk is good for your bones but they neglect to mention the pH process. Calcium mined from the earth and sold in supplement form has been linked to, but not limited to, arthritis and stone formation in the body. The book *The Calcium Lie* by Dr. Robert Thompson, M.D., explains that there are multiple minerals comprising the bones and by focusing primarily on calcium, you are not serving your body well.[3] The process of creating calcium in the body is done through biological transmutation. You'll need magnesium, phosphorus and sulfur included in the dozen or so minerals necessary to create strong bones. By supplementing your diet with high quality unprocessed salt and trace minerals, you'll improve bone density.

Before I leave the subject of milk, I think it's important to note another issue. This issue is the completely misleading industry of *fat free*. When it comes to milk, it has more carbohydrates than protein. Carbohydrates are broken down into sugar in the body, thereby affecting the powerful blood sugar once again. However, the fat in milk actually slows the rate at which sugar is utilized. When you remove the fat from dairy, you'll get a faster burn of sugar, negatively affecting insulin levels. A side effect of the insulin response required to stabilize blood sugar is the production of triglycerides, which factor into obesity.

If you're going to consume dairy, go for the organic whole milk products. If you're interested in upgrading your choices even more, look for quality dairies that supply raw milk. Unpasteurized milk contains enzymes that aid in digestion. Most grocery stores carry organic cheeses made with raw milk products. Pasteurization has killed the enzymes and beneficial bacteria naturally occurring in dairy products. Again, it's important to find quality dairy. You need to be certain the farmer has taken into consideration the ill effects of hormones, antibiotics and toxins in the animals' diet. Ask the farmer if you can tour the dairy and inquire about pharmaceuticals used on the livestock. Personally, I don't drink milk unless it's raw milk I've fermented into kefir.

Returning to the acid/alkaline system, it's useful to note the trace minerals mentioned a few times already will help to reduce the acidity in the body. The 84 trace minerals have a very alkalinizing affect. However, if you subject high quality salt to high heat during the cooking process, you'll destroy minerals. Without these minerals present, salt will have detrimental effects. This is why I suggest adding them to your drinking water. If you cook with high quality salts, be sure to add them at the very last stage of cooking or after the meal has been prepared. Table salt has been processed at over 1,200 degrees Fahrenheit, negatively affecting its chemical structure and destroying the trace minerals.

Earlier, I mentioned kefir. This fermented drink provides beneficial bacteria. This is another very important piece to the digestion puzzle. Beneficial bacteria are also referred to as probiotics. Biotic means life. Pro is *for* and anti is *against*. Many people are suffering systemically because of the indiscriminate elimination of beneficial bacteria due to the overuse of antibiotics. Probiotics aid in digestion and play a major role in proper immune function. Store bought yogurt will have a small amount of bacteria cultures. If you purchase probiotic pills, make sure to buy a refrigerated brand. Fermenting your own probiotic food is an excellent way to repopulate the beneficial bacteria.[4]

When you start to see the big picture, you begin to see why so many people are struggling with poor health, depression and lack of love. The ways in which we care for our bodies is becoming increasingly dis-integrated. Again, before you purchase another supplement, ask yourself how this supplement fits into the body as a whole. Do you have a singular objective in taking this supplement? Do you truly understand how the lack of this supplement affects you holistically?

It is appropriate to address fitness holistically as well. If you measured the amount of nutrients in the body after working only your legs, like you would in weight lifting, you would find the legs received more nutrition. Nutrient delivery correlates with activity. If your only form of working out is dis-integrated into separate days for different segments of the body, you would not be caring for the body as a whole. True health is holistic. It needs to be approached as such. Weight lifting is not bad. It's just that most activities in life, sports or physical recreation require a body that works as a functional whole, not one that has been exclusively trained to work in two-dimensional space, disintegrated. A nice solution would be to add yoga, Pilates or rebounding to compliment your weight lifting regimen. Indian clubs are a great variation for weight bearing fitness to integrate your entire body, three-dimensionally. Exercise is necessary but know that it's stressful on the body. It creates an acid state. It's important to alkalinize your body after exercise.

We should exercise to keep our bodies functional and eat to maintain optimal health. During an interview with Patrick Timpone, Daniel Vitalis pointed out the ineffectiveness of spending money on empty calories, and then spending vast amounts of energy trying to burn off the calories we just ate so we don't gain weight.[5] It's a waste of money, time and effort to consume poor quality food. Instead, it makes more sense to improve the quality of your food and reduce the quantity. If you also improve digestion then you're actually getting more for your money.

The same theory is true for taking trace minerals. Since minerals improve biological function, it stands to reason that all supplements taken could be reduced because now your body is potentially functioning more efficiently. It can also affect the dosage of medication you consume since the body will function at a higher level with trace minerals. Of course you would want to consult with your physician or other health care provider before you decide to adjust prescription dosages. All around, a few shifts in awareness and diet can improve your health and well-being not to mention, save a few dollars.

Your body needs a certain amount of calories per day to run metabolic functions. If you deprive yourself of the calories necessary to run basal processes, your body will not be in harmony. If you eat empty calories, your body will experience a certain amount of stress attempting to assimilate and utilize food that is not natural for our species. Many grocery store shelves are filled with products that look like food but they're seen as foreign substances within our bodies.

There are many studies showing the effects of unhealthy food choices on our emotions and states of mind. Intoxicants such as alcohol can have more immediate effects but the subtle effects of hormone dysfunction from alcohol can be harder to recognize. Drinking alcohol with meals will hinder digestion. Without proper digestion, the hormone serotonin is not adequately produced. This hormone contributes to feelings of happiness. Serotonin functions in relation to melatonin, which helps us to sleep effectively.

Disruptions in digestion and hormone regulation affect cortisol levels, which have a wide range of effects in the body from the storage of fat to thyroid dysfunction and stress. The thyroid is one of the first systems of defense in the body. It works in relationship to cortisol. Picture a steering wheel that needs to be turned with two hands. Cortisol supplies one hand and thyroid hormones supply the other. If you over stimulate cortisol throughout your life, it may take its hand off the wheel eventually. This inefficiency will affect energy levels and metabolic activity. Read about nascent iodine for supporting the thyroid.

It's important to address your habits and find out how they're affecting your overall happiness. It's okay to occasionally consume alcohol, eat empty calories or experience stress, but if this is your way of life, you will need to make some upgrades if you want to activate more of genetic potential. If you want to thrive, you should stop using the microwave. Dr. Mercola wrote a very compelling article on the dangers of this appliance. During his review of many studies conducted on food preparation with a microwave, he stated, "The apparently toxic effects of microwave cooking is another in a long list of unnatural additives in our daily diets."[6] Microwaved food is barely recognizable to our bodies. It takes more energy to utilize food that has been overcooked, microwaved or highly processed. Do you feel you have adequate energy to throw away on poor food choices? The real question is which came first, the low energy or the inferior food?

Trace minerals and B vitamins will increase your energy. If you mix B vitamins with antioxidants you increase their effectiveness even more. Vitamin C helps with depression, fatigue and fat loss. Again, it's imperative you obtain a bioavailable source for your vitamins and minerals. David Wolfe claims that when you add probiotics to the vitamins and minerals listed above, you increase their effectiveness once again. Wolfe is featured in multiple documentaries, has written several books and provides quality supplements at *Longevity Warehouse*. Vitamins and minerals ideally need to come from your food. Whole food supplements are more readily absorbed and utilized. Cheap supplements are mostly made from synthetics and are not easily recognized by your body. Most of these materials are released in your urine within hours of consuming if your processes of elimination are functioning as they should. If you are not able to excrete these materials, you may end up storing them in your tissues. Lately, people have been telling me they've heard vitamins are not proven to improve your health. If the people in the study were on medications or do not have their DAUX systems functioning effectively, they may not benefit from supplements. If the vitamins were not made from whole foods, then they may not prove to be beneficial.

You will replace millions of cells today throughout your vast, interwoven system. Now is the time to activate your potential and rebuild your cells with love, positive thoughts and adequate nutrition. With a holistic view, you have the potential to be more than the sum of your parts. Reductionist thinking removes responsibility from the consequences of our actions in relation to our bodies and our environments. It is time to improve our *response-ability* with a high regard for the world in which we live.

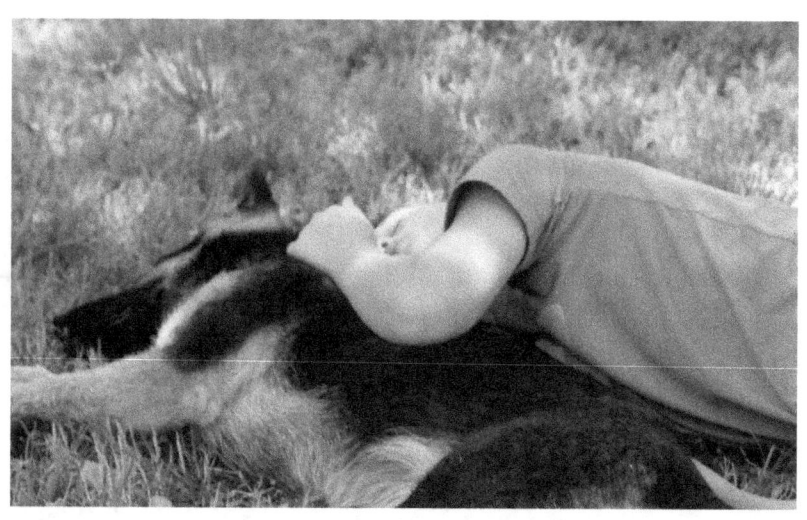

You may say I'm a dreamer, but I'm not the only one.
I hope someday you'll join us. And the world will live as one.
John Lennon

CHAPTER 8

RECIPE FOR AWAKENING

Every great dream begins with a dreamer.
Always remember, you have within you the
strength, the patience, and the passion to reach
for the stars to change the world.
Harriet Tubman

Every morning, awaken spiritually, physically and mentally. Many people miss these opportunities each day and are not fully awake to the world around them. Make an effort to wake up naturally, without an alarm. Breathe in the awareness of self-love and take a moment to recall your dreams. Due to the ephemeral nature of dreams, they are fragile and easily lost. Therefore, before you engage in thoughts, try to record your dreams. Recollect as much information as you can, writing down the major symbols, people and feelings associated with the actions.

Many people claim they don't remember their dreams. The first step in recalling your dreams is to *decide* to remember your dreams. Secondly, you'll need a notebook to record their messages. Throughout my life, I've been told to keep a notebook by my bed so I can record my dreams in case I wake up in the middle of the night. Usually, I wait until morning. Many times, memory of a dream will be triggered during the day. Write these down as well. You can come up with creative ideas, find lost objects and solve problems in dreams, just to name a few themes. If the dream doesn't trigger everyday understanding, look into symbolism to provide another perspective. Some dreams are clearly meaningful while others are considered to be fragmented images from a hectic life. Some methods of analysis can hijack your dream so it's important to allow the feelings of the dream to guide you. Consult multiple dream analysis books to see what methods appeal to you. I personally enjoy the *Dreamer's Dictionary* published by The School of Metaphysics.[1] Dreams have insightful and profound messages to guide you on your journey. I strongly believe dreams provide keys to our spiritual evolution. You spend one third of your life sleeping and dreaming. This alone is meaningful and worthy of your attention. Once you make a conscious effort to remember your dreams, you may be surprised at how much information they contain.

The mental and physical benefits of sleeping and dreaming are vast. Dr. Rubin Naiman, Ph.D., sleep and dream specialist, claims, "We don't get sleep because we don't *get* sleep."[2] If we fully understood the purpose of sleeping and dreaming, we would raise our level of care concerning these functions in our lives. We greatly hinder the benefits of these processes by drinking alcohol or taking sleeping pills at bedtime. In order to aid in natural sleep, start by taking one milligram of melatonin nightly. Taking melatonin will not interfere with your body's ability to make melatonin. Watching television until you fall asleep, being exposed to unnatural light or excessive electromagnetic fields in the bedroom will contribute to poor quality sleep. Consequently, cellular regeneration and the intuition gained from dreaming is also diminished under these conditions. Consider sleeping with a grounding sheet from The Earthing Company. Use an eye pillow. Restrict television use an hour before bedtime. Soften the lights or consider using candles during this time and do some deep breathing exercises. Read about the benefits of herbs like chamomile, lavender or valerian for better sleep.

The neurotransmitter serotonin is converted into melatonin at night. If you have a deficiency in one of these transmitters, you most likely have a deficiency in the other. Serotonin is related to feelings of happiness and well-being. It's linked with the forebrain and is produced mainly in the digestive system. You may have already started to realize how your happiness and your ability to sleep soundly are woven together and are directly related to your nutrition. A lack of sleep will increase cortisol levels throughout the day. By spiking these levels during the day, you affect your ability to fully regenerate during the sleep cycle. This near constant state of stress we create for our bodies affects our minds. During this state we are mostly responding to life in the survival modes of fight, flight or freeze. If you consider the laws of attraction in this scenario, being in stress attracts stress. At the very least, it contributes to how you view and react to the world around you.

After recalling your dreams in the morning, bring your awareness back to self-love. Take a few moments to follow your breath, becoming aware of your body in the present. In the beginning, you may need to repeat a mantra to keep your attention focused on your love of self. Ultimately, you will not want to associate your love with anything or anyone in particular. It will predominantly be a feeling maintained in a state of no-thought.

After you have awakened to heightened awareness through the breath, shift your attention to your body. A considerable amount of energy was needed for rebuilding and cleansing during the night. While you've slept, it was helpful for your body not to have its resources devoted to digestion, which also takes a tremendous amount of energy. Your blood sugar has dropped and will need to be stimulated in order to keep your body out of stress. Mineral and enzyme deficiencies will also need to be addressed at the start of the day. Minerals are necessary for enzymes to function. Enzymes run all of the processes in your body.

If you prioritize your day according to your basic survival needs, the following requirement will be water. If you want to upgrade beyond surviving to thriving, have the BodyMind morning drink suggested in Chapter 4. This drink will assist with cell function, stabilize blood sugar and aid in cleansing. A half a cup of juice will be in your bloodstream in five minutes to stimulate your blood sugar and give you some energy. (Allow this drink at least five minutes to empty your stomach before you have breakfast.) A full glass of juice will over stimulate this process, creating stress in your body. Remember that cortisol is produced during times of stress. There are many side effects to over production of cortisol: adrenal fatigue, thyroid issues, belly-fat, not to mention its effect on your state of mind. If you drink coffee before water and minerals, you'll create disharmony in your body. Unfortunately, this is so common for some people that they have acclimated to the stimulation of coffee and no longer recognize this as stress. Don't let this blind you to its effects.

You may interpret stress as a boost to get moving. At times, cortisol production is a means to escape from trouble. However, if one doesn't escape from trouble and metabolize the stress hormones on the brain, this will cause problems. Their cumulative effects will damage or kill brain cells over time. One method of escape is running. However, this response was mainly intended for short bursts; it was not intended for us to run from trouble for miles and miles, every day. Remember that vigorous exercise, regardless of its positive effects, is stressful on the body. You will need to cultivate a lifestyle of rapidly delivering your body to a calm state after a stressful event.

According to Ray Peat, who holds a Ph.D. in Biology, coffee can be a healthy drink if you add cream and sugar. Ideally, upgrade to organic or raw cream and a high quality, natural sweetener like yakon, honey or agave. This combination will reduce the stimulant effects of coffee, putting less strain on your adrenal system. It's beneficial to drink a cup of coffee slowly to reduce the effect on the adrenals.[3] Coffee is heavily sprayed with pesticides so make an effort to buy organic brands. Dave Asprey informs the public that the mycotoxins produced from the mold in coffee, even organic brands, causes many of its detrimental effects. Roasting coffee can kill the mold but not the toxins the mold emits. His Bulletproof® Coffee addresses these toxins. He suggests that you add MCT oil (a derivative of coconut oil) and unsalted grass-fed butter to his upgraded coffee for optimal brain function, healthy weight and a cascade of other benefits.[4]

Let's get back to your awakened morning. Because you've had the splash of juice in your mineral water, your blood sugar has been stimulated and is hopefully low and even. If you skip the morning drink and fix a typical breakfast, you will put strain on your body as it waits for food to be digested and delivered to your bloodstream for energy conversion. Considering gastric empty times, it will take over an hour for a typical breakfast to make its way through your digestive system. Even if you eat a high quality breakfast, your body will be anxious if it has to wait the hour or more for the sugar to equalize your system. This lack of blood sugar stabilization will cause cortisol production as the body accesses stored glucose for energy. The morning drink will avert the stress response while your breakfast works its way through the system. If you skip both the morning drink *and* breakfast, you will create even more tension in your body. Again, some people have become so accustomed to this troubled state; they no longer recognize it as stress. It's just life.

While you've slept, your body was cleansing waste from your cells. This waste has been emptied from your cells like trash on the streets. Your lymph system will need to cleanse this debris from your body. However, the lymph is a pump-less system and it will need your assistance. Think of exercise as a street sweeper. Try doing a few minutes of yoga to pump the lymph system. The best types of exercise for pumping the lymph system are rebounding, yoga and Pilates. These forms of fitness work the body as a whole. They do not separate or dis-integrate the body. They are also considered, non-impact. Therefore, before you have breakfast, it's suggested to pump your lymph system for five minutes with an integrated, non-impact method of fitness while keeping your focus on your breath.

I know many people would say they don't have time for a morning like this. So far, my suggestions have only taken about 15 minutes. Attempt to sleep earlier or wake up earlier. Do whatever it takes to honor your extraordinary existence; the positive effects are worth it. If you are married or sleep with a significant other, an awakened morning would be a perfect way to honor your relationship. Try partner yoga. It's a wonderful modality to connect with your love and learn about one another on a subtle level. If you have children, tend to your needs first whenever possible. Think of the oxygen mask on the airplane. This recipe for awakening would be nice for your children as well. In the event of babies that possibly need immediate attention or some other unexpected event that occurs, try to return to a quiet place for yourself before you get too busy. Everyone you encounter will benefit from your stress-free presence.

Additionally, be mindful of gastric empty times before completing a full exercise regimen. After a meal, your blood needs to be in your core to aid in digestion. When you exercise, your blood will flow to your extremities. Allow time for digestion if you want to keep your body out of stress. Poor digestion affects absorption of nutrients, which then affects utilization of nutrients, as well as excretion of waste. A general timeline for digestion is listed in Appendix II. If you're limited on time for fitness, rebounding is an excellent choice. Five minutes on a rebounder is equivalent to 20 minutes of traditional cardiovascular exercise. This non-impact method exercises every cell in the body and assists with excretion of waste. (Note: It's important to select a quality rebounder. Visit www.mindmirror.org for recommendations.) It's always effective to diversify your workout. Try dancing for cardio periodically. This is a great way to pump the lymph system and integrate whole body movement. For isometric exercise, repeatedly contract your muscles for six seconds and release. This simple method could be done at a desk, in your car or on a plane. When you exercise be present with yourself and feel love.

Make a conscious effort to begin each day with promise, gratitude and awareness. Activate more of your genetic potential with proper nutrition and peace of soul. Today is a *renew* day. Prioritize it in accordance with vitality and mastery. Operate from essence as you follow your dreams.

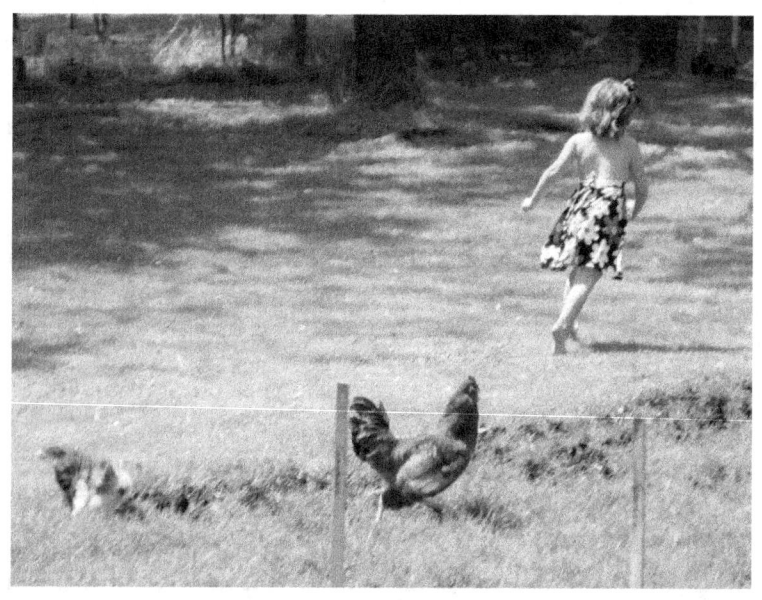

One touch of nature makes the whole world kin.

William Shakespeare

CHAPTER 9

SOMETIMES NEGATIVITY IS A GOOD THING

*And forget not that the earth delights to feel your bare feet
and the winds long to play with your hair.*
Kahlil Gibran *The Prophet*

Our lives are lived increasingly indoors. It's imperative we go outside to achieve greater harmony in our lives. We need negative ions to clean the air, lift our mood and aid in healing. Per cubic centimeter fresh mountain or country air could have around 30-40,000 negative ions. In the city, there is a decrease of 10-20,000. Inside a building you might find negative ions will be as low as 1000 negative ions per cubic centimeter. If the city is very polluted the ions inside could drop to 100. When you stand next to a waterfall or walk on a beach, you could find ions in the range of 100,000 per cubic centimeter.[1] Ions also increase after rain or a storm. It would be beneficial to go outside and do deep breathing after a rainstorm. Negative ions activate positive hormones, including but not limited to serotonin, insulin and melatonin. Negative ions also assist with nutrient delivery. Take time to visit places that provide these ions. To increase negative ions inside, you could use a salt lamp or purchase a negative ionizer. The sun gives off positive radiation. From the beginning of time, we have been in direct contact with the earth to provide the negative electrons necessary to counter this radiation. In the natural health community, we call this direct (skin to earth) connection, *grounding*. Unfortunately, modern life has led us indoors. According to David Wolfe, the worst invention of our time is shoes. They disconnect us from the earth and the unnatural phenomenon of wearing shoes has contributed to many health detriments. He even discusses a correlation between wearing shoes and Multiple Sclerosis (MS). He believes one of the best things you can do for MS is to walk barefoot on the beach, close to the shore, on a sunny day.[2]

At one point in history, people slept on the earth. Now, we are inside or in shoes for the majority of our lives. This disconnection from the earth has led to a lack of reverence for our planet. It has also contributed to the lack of negative electrons in our body. These electrons contribute to healing and are necessary in preventing free radicals from destroying healthy tissue. Most people have heard about free radicals and their widespread destruction. The free radical process is a system to remove dead or dying cells. Free radicals are positively charged molecules short of one electron. They are emitted from cells to help destroy harmful microorganisms and damaged tissue. Free radicals steal electrons from damaged cells preparing them for disposal from the body. When the cells have been removed, ideally, the body will have free electrons available to stabilize this molecule and bring this cycle to a healthy stopping point. Unfortunately, this noble mission can lead to chronic inflammation if the body lacks the necessary electrons needed to effectively bring the free radical process to a close.[3]

It's possible for you to gain the free electrons you're missing from antioxidants. However, due to insufficient nutrition, these electron donors are lacking as well. At this point in our history, we're going to need all of the help we can get. Walking barefoot on the earth is a beneficial method to gain these electrons. For some, this option has been greatly diminished. Thankfully, there is technology from The Earthing Company that can assist with electron deficiency. This technology can limit the harmful effects of electromagnetic fields, as well as provide free electrons by simulating a direct connection to the earth. I sleep with this technology and use their grounding mats when I'm going to be spending extended periods at the computer. The best way however, is to spend time daily, outside, connected barefoot to the earth.

Spending time outdoors is the ideal way to get vitamin D. We obtain this important nutrient from sunlight and some foods. Vitamin D plays a role in various biological processes from weight loss to immune function. This unique vitamin is turned into a hormone inside your body and its role is vital to many organs, strong bones, respiration and brain development. During the winter months, it is recommended that you supplement with a high quality vitamin D3 from a reputable supplier.

Consider your daily routine. How much of it is spent indoors breathing stagnant air, exposed to electro magnetic fields and subjected to unnatural light? Use your breaks wisely. Opt for sunshine, fresh air and grounding.

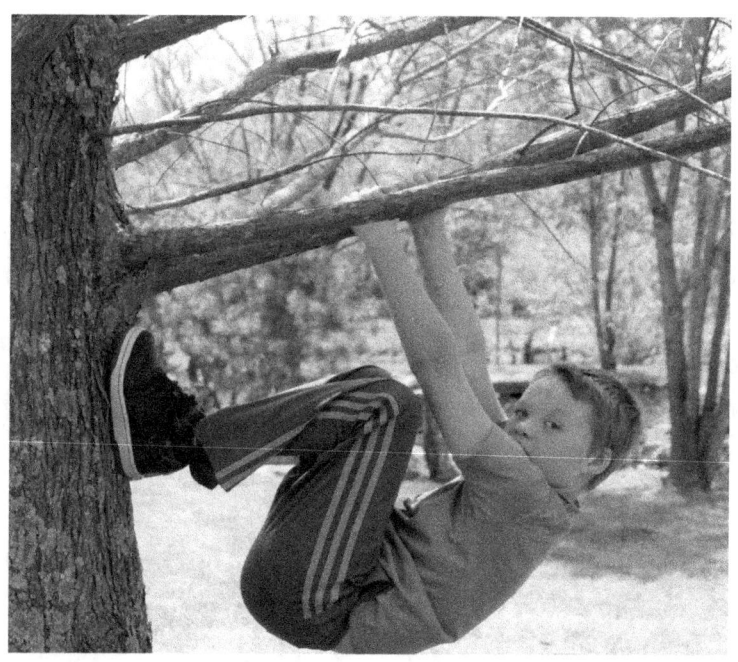

Only when the last tree has died and the last river has been poisoned
and the last fish been caught will we realize we cannot eat money.
Cree Proverb

CHAPTER 10

BEYOND LIMITED BELIEF

Once you realize the interconnectedness of your body,
you start to see patterns connecting you to all of life.
When you take responsibility for your life you take
responsibility for all of life.
Paul Williams *Das Energi*

Just as we consume vast amounts of water that never reaches the interior of the cell and we eat food that mystifies our bodies' biological processes, we seek love outside of ourselves, preventing true growth. We turn to others to feel love and too often we focus on keeping our relationships alive instead of ourselves. In times of loss and struggle, we have the most opportunity to learn the power and beauty of higher consciousness. Yet it's often during these times that we disconnect from spirit and turn to medication, poor food choices or other people to remove the pain. This is equivalent to fruit that is picked before it's ripe. We are disconnecting from the source without a sense of completeness. This affects our ability to be truly happy when alone or in relationships. When we move further and further away from self-reliance, be that emotionally or in our food supply, the closer we get to dependency.

When we depend on others for our happiness and for our food, we put our health in the hands of others. It only takes a slight amount of investigation to realize you can't always trust food that has origins unknown to you. With all of the misinformation in our minds, it's difficult enough to know ourselves, let alone truly know another. Why would we put our happiness in someone's hands before we have true understanding of who they are? How can we expect to see who someone is if we can't even see ourselves? When we remove the toxins in our minds and bodies, we will see more clearly and our relationships will truly prosper. By putting your health in the doctor's hands, you are admitting you don't know your own body or how it functions. I believe it's important to become your own primary care provider. It's possible to learn enough about your bodily functions and nutrition to make wiser decisions about your health. It will be one of the best investments of your time you've ever made.

There are no guarantees you'll restore perfect health but I feel confident saying you'll improve your chances, beyond limited belief. I've seen multiple documentaries and have read countless stories about people who have overcome grave illnesses with proper nutrition and natural protocols. If your life is being acutely threatened by disease, it may be a risky move to rely on nature verses western medicine. I certainly wouldn't want to be faced with that decision. If you were given a terminal diagnosis and you found out your condition could possibly have been prevented if you had taken in proper nutrition, how would you feel? Would you wish you could turn back the clock so you didn't have to face the choice of radical procedure verses natural protocols? If you are *not* faced with a terminal illness, pretend you're turning back the clock now and be diligent with your health as if your life depended on it, because it does.

Just as some people think they're loving themselves, most people think they're eating a healthy diet. Being a nutritionist, I often hear people say their nutrition isn't bad but it doesn't take long for me to see the misinformation they've been relying on to be healthy. You qualify for an upgrade, especially if you're taking prescription medications. When it comes to acute, critical care, our doctors are heroes. Unfortunately, our health care system has turned to chronic sick care. Medicine has become specialized instead of holistic. If you continue to truncate and treat symptoms without a holistic viewpoint, your results will certainly fall short of your expectations.

For over a decade, I've been advising people on nutrition. In the beginning, the information I shared came from mainstream sources and I've since discovered there is a lot of misinformation and propaganda surrounding our food supply. It's hard to know who is selling something beneficial and who has paid for their market share. For this reason, I gather the majority of my knowledge from people who are living healthy lives in harmony with nature. In order to be naturally healthy, one must follow the advice of experts in the field of natural health.

During the last several years, I've felt privileged to study with experts in the field of natural health. The information I've put forth in this book will hopefully give you a baseline for returning your body to optimal health. I have not spent time on specific, day-to-day meal planning. Instead, I wanted to present a perspective of holism and encourage you to investigate the diet that is right for you. I have mentioned many people I consider to be credible in the field of nutrition. Consult their books, listen to their interviews online or hire a BodyMind Nutritionist to guide you towards self-mastery.

New information becomes available frequently; therefore, you will want to be diligent about continuing your health education. New documentaries about our food supply are being released regularly. Some of the films I've listed in Appendix II are a few years old but I recommend watching them if you haven't already. Discerning good information from bad will be easier if you spend time learning about the trivium. The trivium consists of grammar, logic and rhetoric.[1] This method of reasoning will prove invaluable to you. Our critical thinking skills are being systematically removed from our education, hindering our self-reliance. Merging the trivium with Nonviolent Communication will promote healthier dialog in your relationships.[2]

One shouldn't be dismayed at changing nutritional advice. When it comes to new information, you must drift like a cloud and flow like water. Many foods once touted as beneficial have proven to have detrimental effects due to genetic modification. For this reason, I've included a link to OrganicConsumers.Org to learn about the effects of genetically engineered food. They make it easy to get involved in order to change the political landscape of food production.[3] You can take a stand every time you sit down to eat and it begins by voting with your dollars at the grocery store. Improvement of the general food supply increases your chances of mastery. If everyone upgraded their choices and shifted their perspective towards vitality, we would all benefit.

Don't allow your education to become stagnant by hanging on to outdated beliefs. Most of the grocery store shelves are stocked with companies that receive an F rating in the *Better World Shopper.* Our bodies are fairly forgiving. Many people have been eating a highly processed, microwaved, pesticide laden diet for years and appear to be healthy. Therefore, if you have been eating GMO food or if other advice you once trusted has proven to be invalid, you'll most likely recover with some awareness, discipline and upgrades to your diet.

I often hear people claim it's too difficult to remember all of this information or they don't have time to study what is right for them. Realistically, the information is quite simple once you understand the whys of making the transition to more natural food. Daniel Vitalis suggests we concentrate on eating like our species would. He reminds us that you won't find Doritos or Chips Ahoy growing in nature.[4] Nature also provides us with many cures for common ailments. Keep in mind; our bodies are deficient in minerals not pharmaceuticals. Michael Pollan, author of *In Defense of Food*, humorously suggests this, "If it comes from a plant, eat it; if it was made in a plant, don't."

I've heard people say they don't have the money to eat quality food. Take time to consider the unnecessary purchases you've made before you settle on this excuse. In many instances it's a matter of priorities; other times it's a lack of education. You've heard the phrase: "If you give a man a fish, you feed him for an evening but when you teach a man to fish, you feed him for a lifetime." With this in mind, know that our food welfare system is definitely in need of upgrades. Soda, white bread, sweets and chips, just to name a few, should not be allowed. Are we really doing the best we can to help care for our poor, or rather, help them to care for themselves? It's also important to note corporations are profiting from producing cheap unhealthy food that is subsidized by our tax dollars. You're paying in advance for low quality food and you'll pay later with poor health.

To disassociate from poor food choices, I suggest people take a healthy lunch and nutritious snacks to work. People claim they don't have time in the morning to prepare healthy food. You will have to make food a priority. Without your health, you cannot fully enjoy your family, work, hobbies or material possessions. If you or one of your family members were faced with a life-threatening illness, how would your priorities shift? Some say their spouses and children don't want to change the way they eat. Are these satisfactory reasons for not taking control of your health and happiness? There are no magical solutions. It's time to take control of your life and you'll be rewarded in countless ways.

I say this with great confidence, if you give your body what it needs to thrive and tune your mind towards love, a happier, more peaceful life will unfold before you. A mind and body returned to harmony will intrinsically know and feel what it's been missing. I believe we are genetically coded to naturally experience extraordinary states, currently unknown to most of us. We have the capacity to be more than we are. Often times, our ambitions are materialistic instead of spiritualistic. I believe our standards for health and love are set too low.

Nutritional recommendations are mostly based on studies of subjects who are not healthy, let alone functioning at their optimal potential. If your body doesn't assimilate nutrients efficiently, you will have deficiencies. You may find current suggestions for food quantity would be much less if your body adequately utilized what you've consumed. If we focused on eating more nutrient dense superfood smoothies for breakfast, we could reduce the portion size of subsequent meals. Your brain function may exceed your expectations and current understanding of the world, given superior nutrition.

All medical, dietetic, wellness and scientific data has been conducted using participants who have NOT been first fully calibrated with a system that would restore their full electrical, mineral, hydration, nutrient, detoxification and DAUX (Digestion, Absorption, Utilization and eXcretion) capacity.

Lars Gustafsson founder of The BodyMind Institute

The Recommended Daily Allowance (RDA) is primarily based on preventing deficiency diseases not preventing chronic diseases nor is it focused on achieving optimum health. Until we honestly treat ourselves to very best holistic care, how will we ever know what our potential is? I believe when we reach mastery, we won't need a food pyramid to tell us what to eat; our intuition will guide us. With a high regard for yourself as a sentient, sapient being, you will be able to highly regard the world around you. When we demonstrate respect for all living things, true knowledge and true love will surround us.

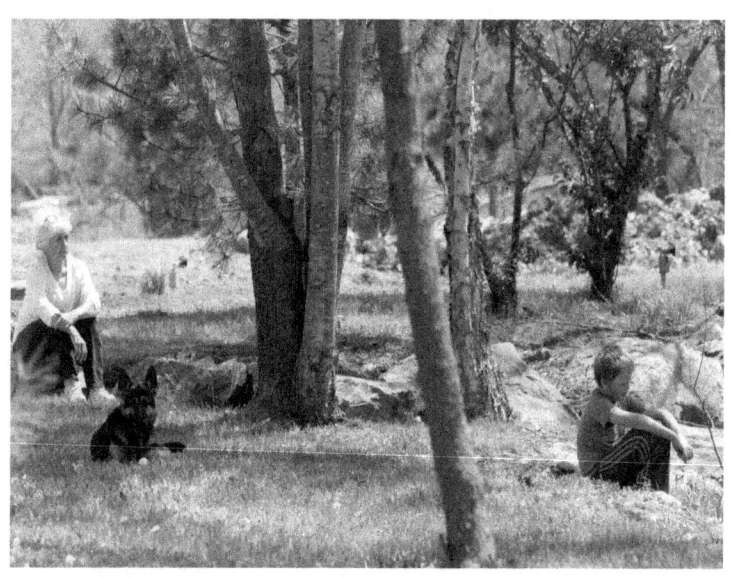

How far you go in life depends on your being tender with the young, compassionate with the aged, sympathetic with the striving and tolerant of the weak and strong. Because someday in your life you will have been all of these.

George Washington Carver

CHAPTER 11

PEACE OF THE PUZZLE

Every conquering temptation represents a new fund of moral energy.
Every trial endured and weathered in the right spirit makes a
soul nobler and stronger than it was before.
William Butler Yeats

You need a certain amount of energy to be grounded, peaceful and connected to the power of the present moment. However, if you're allowing your energy to be depleted with resentment, jealousy, greed, attachment, etc. you're creating a state of disharmony in your presence. When you give more energy to your past than to your present, you're missing out on life. When you spend time gossiping about others, you're allowing your subtle peaceful energy to leave your body. Peace and disharmony are mutually exclusive. You cannot maintain both states simultaneously.

The next time you're feeling somewhat pessimistic or seem to be in a negative mood, take the time to consider what your nutrition was like for the last 24 hours. Potentially, you have subtly sent your body into stress, which has shifted your perspective towards survival. Be gentle with yourself. Breathe deeply and center yourself in a loving, forgiving place. After five deep breaths, you should feel better. Even if the stress your body is experiencing is subtle, you will not be functioning at your optimal level. You will not reach your genetic and spiritual potential in disharmony. If your body and mind are in states of survival or protection, you will not be in a state of growth. Bruce Lipton, Ph.D., in his book *Spontaneous Evolution*, notes a study where cells in a Petri dish will open and move towards nutrients. When a toxin is presented, the cell will close and move away from the toxin. He states, "A cell cannot be in a state of growth and a state of protection at the same time."[1]

If you're protecting yourself through isolation, hanging on to negative emotions or criticizing others, you will not be in a state of growth. Our bodies and spirits are meant to live in harmony. The fight or flight systems are for those *just in case* moments. Yet how many of us are living our days in these states, constantly? We are meant to live in harmony with nature but how many times a day are our actions linked with the good of the planet? How many times a day are we supporting big corporations that get F's in environmental and social responsibility? Examine your purchases from toothpaste to cars. Are you making a positive difference with every dollar you spend or are you contributing to greed, corruption and destruction by financially supporting F companies? We're meant to live in harmony with one another but how many people are we hurting because we're not dedicated to self-mastery? How many of us have stopped far short of our genetic potential and spiritual brilliance?

How many fabrications do we tell ourselves to justify our lifestyles? Don Miguel Ruiz, author of *The Fifth Agreement*, tells us, "Our dream is controlled by what we believe, and what we believe could be truth, or could be fiction. The truth leads us to our authenticity, to happiness. Lies lead us to limitations in our lives, to suffering and drama."[2] Our opinions about ourselves and our opinions about others are not necessarily true. Until we tune into the subtle energy of our bodies, we will continue to tune out the truth of who we are.

Now, more than ever, it is vital we reconnect with our essence and raise our standards of personal interaction to a new level. John Maxwell Taylor, a pioneer in *Transformational Theater*, expressed that the majority of the people you will interact with today or any given day are disembodied and will steal your energy to empower themselves. They have lost touch with their spirit and no longer connect with people in meaningful ways. Many people operate from personality instead of essence.[3] If our personalities are fabrications based on misconceptions how can we be living an authentic life? If we don't realize many of our motivations are misguided, how can we truly be happy? I like to think that innately we are all good. However, if we are selling ourselves counterfeit beliefs, we will never redeem our amazing potential.

The depletion of our natural resources and polluting of our air so we can manufacture material goods to pacify our longings is not sustainable. Depletion of our energy and vital functions through alcohol, drugs or other toxic habits is not sustainable. Sure, we can get by for a while. We're highly resilient, but why not use our resilience to detoxify and heal verses using it to further contaminate our planet and ourselves? I've read countless spiritual books, taken transformative workshops and immersed myself in teachings on the human potential movement. However, if I didn't practice the teachings daily to maintain a new level of existence, I found myself depleted, time and time again. To make lasting change, it takes continuous effort. But don't be dismayed at the word "effort". Attempting an awakened state of peace is more rewarding than accepting unhappiness and pain.

I don't lead an impeccable life, completely free from bad habits and sadness. However, I believe any effort I put towards a more sustainable and peaceful future will make a difference. There is a story of a boy walking near the ocean. The tide had come in and left 1000's of starfish stranded on the beach. The boy began throwing the starfish, one by one, back into the sea. A witness came along and said, "I'm afraid you're not going to make a difference, young man. These stranded starfish go on for miles." The boy picked up another starfish, throwing it back into the water, and said, "I bet it will make a difference to this one." Like the boy, I believe our positive contributions matter. There are many times we will waver, nutritionally and spiritually but we shouldn't let those times take us completely off course.

If you're feeling lost and unhappy, the true way is there. It's more satisfying, real and alive than any experience you can imagine. Poet David Whyte expressed, "You will know that you are on the right way if the road totally disappears. You know that you are doing something radical because you can't see where you're going. Everything that you have lent on for your identity has gone. And you will enter the black, contemplative splendors of self-doubt at the same time that you are setting out on this new radical path."[4] Stillness and a quiet mind are the first steps to finding your way again. It takes a courageous and adventurous spirit to brave the dark woods alone. Yet if you don't know you are lost, you will continue to bolster your self-esteem and net-worth struggling to find peace. To quote from another poet David Waggoner in his work *Lost,* he stated, "Stand still. The trees ahead and bushes beside you are not lost... The forest knows where you are. You must let it find you."[5]

Connecting with nature is a wonderful way to reconnect with yourself. Sit barefoot in the grass, listening to the sounds, feeling the wind and smelling the scents of nature. Attempt to maintain a state of *no thought* but total presence of yourself. To feel your entire body while in tune with your surroundings, aware of the observer within you is true power. Conducting yourself with this sort of presence may be fairly natural in a garden or on a secluded beach but once you enter the crowded city or hectic work environment, you may find yourself lost again. It becomes increasingly important to embody your total being. Learn techniques to bring yourself fully into the moment and reenergize your spirit.

In my yoga classes, I teach students a grounding exercise. I have them close their eyes while standing and feel both feet. They observe whether they are putting more weight in the left or right foot. Then I have them subtly shift to the right then to the left. I suggest they shift from front to back, placing more weight in the heels and then the toes. Eventually, they position themselves evenly on both feet with equal emphasis from front to back. I have them follow this awareness throughout their bodies, stopping at major landmarks. The process takes about a minute. When they open their eyes, they are stoic and still. They appear to be stronger, centered and fully present. They tell me they can feel the shift in their awareness, every time.

This grounding exercise is great if you have a minute. If you're caught off guard and need to compose yourself in an instant, you could intently bring your attention to your feet, legs or hands to center your attention on your body. During times of meditation, I may have people focus on their heart center and breathe deeply while emanating a loving feeling towards themselves. However, if you're taken by surprise or fear and your heart is pounding, this may not be the place to send your attention. Try breathing into your toes or fingers to take attention off the rapid heartbeat. When you're more calm, return to your heart center.

Sometimes it's useful to give yourself affirmations. When framing your suggestions affirm the positive instead of the negative. You can't say, *I don't want to be unhappy*. The mind will register the word *unhappy*. It's like saying: *don't picture a red balloon*. Most likely, your mind will see the balloon without registering the word: *don't*. Therefore, affirm that you are happy. Frame affirmations in the present tense. For example, state, *I am happy* versus *I want to be happy*. Strive for a state of *being* not *wanting*. To bring your awareness and presence into sharper focus, breath deeply into your heels and affirm you are powerful and fully loved. Every now and then it's beneficial to visualize your goals. See them in a state of completion, and then imagine yourself in scenarios after having reached your goals. Living in accordance with your dreams becomes much easier when you believe and feel they are real. Sometimes, we need a little extra motivation to align our consciousness with our aspirations. Once you feel the inspiration, it's imperative to take action towards your dreams.

When things seem to be the most difficult, focusing on positive feelings and breathing deeply into the moment may appear to be impossible. During times of heartache or deep sadness, the pain wells up inside you. You may feel like crying is the only option. It's similar to holding your breath too long and you want to collapse into your exhale. Allow the tears to come. They won't last forever. Tears are another way your body cleanses. Chemicals build up in the body during times of stress and tears are one way your body releases these toxins and waste material.

Prolonged thoughts of the past take energy away from creating solutions in the present. Additionally, the vast amount of misinformation will be difficult to navigate. Giving more attention to what's happened instead of what's happening is like trying to use exhaust fumes to power an engine. The fumes are the byproduct.

Your thoughts about *what happened* are what you leave behind, especially since your thoughts about what happened are most likely incorrect. Instead, you need fuel for the engine: forward thinking, inspiration, meditation and positive action.

Meditation guides you into a state of calm awareness. In the last few minutes of my yoga class, during relaxation, I sometimes tell the class this is not the time to fall asleep. This is the time to fall awake to a new awareness of themselves. For many people, the relaxation portion of class is when the thoughts return. When this happens, take a deep breath and let them go back out to sea like a wave leaving the shore. Yes, they will come back like the tide. At times, it's a gentle, low tide washing over your mind softly and you can experience this without being pulled out to sea. Sometimes your thoughts crash back in with great force. Whatever happens, don't let them take you away without total awareness. Become the observer. Don't analyze, diagnose or evaluate what you're feeling or thinking, just listen. In the event the waves are too powerful and you lose your footing, you mustn't struggle. Alan Watts, during a lecture on Zen, said that you couldn't learn to swim by clutching the water. You need to relax and become one with it and then you'll discover you can float.[6]

When problems arise, strive to reach a peaceful place in your mind then consider possible solutions. During college, I worked at a restaurant as a waitress. Some nights, things would start going wrong. Food wouldn't be coming out right, patrons might keep me at the table too long or maybe I would drop and break something. We had a saying for when you were overwhelmed and you weren't able to handle your area on your own. You would calmly go in the back and tell your fellow employees you are *in the weeds*. Next thing you know, people are asking you what you need. They want to know what they can do for you. They don't want you to sit down and talk about all of the things that went wrong. There's no time for that. You need to delegate and they will help pick up the slack. It's forward motion.

How many nights have you gone to sleep struggling with a problem and when you wake up in the morning, for a few moments the pains of the previous day are gone? You don't recall the details. But what do you do next? You recreate it all in your thoughts and you're in the weeds again. Instead, take this time to fuel your next move, your next forward steps. I don't believe it's an accident we wake up feeling clear. It's a hint that today is a new day. It's another chance to create the life you want. If it gets overwhelming, ask for help from people in the flow of creativity. Edwin Louis Cole tells us, "You don't drown by falling in the water; you drown by staying there."

However, you must remember, we're all in this together. I'm not negating individualism or implying we should conduct ourselves like a school of fish. I'm suggesting we raise our awareness, our consciousness to a state honoring the highest course of action for human life. Interdependence verses dependence is key. Our lives are so vastly different that we need a common denominator. My vote goes for Earth. It's the basis for our survival; it's the most significant connection we all share.

I've been around a lot of inspired people and they generally want to use their creativity and resources for the greater good. Initially, it's monetized. For now, money is necessary to transform our world; I strongly believe it won't always be this way. In the meantime, we will need money to restore balance and peace on earth. The other night, I made up a story for my five-year-old niece. It began with her getting the power to create the life she wanted and buy anything she desired. After she had lots of new things, I could tell she lost a little interest. When the story expanded to include giving to others, she became inspired and creative. At that point, she took over the telling of the story. It's natural when our needs or desires are met, we want to reach out and give to others.

In this new awareness, we need to devise a plan to provide for those who can't meet their basic needs. If we're all in this together, we need to throw out a life preserver to those who are sinking. Then we need to provide them with the tools and inspiration to become self-reliant. We need to give a hand-up periodically but not handouts, indefinitely. If enough people become aware of their potential and adequately nourish themselves, we can alter the course of politics to redirect funds to sustainably support life on this planet. We are accepting defeat if we are not part of the flow of positive action to create an inspired world. The miscreants of society are not connected with abundance. They are malnourished, they believe the lies of their story and they feel they need to steal, harm or destroy in order to survive. This is based on faulty beliefs and a brain in stress. It's hard to dismantle these beliefs when you are hungry, struggling to keep the lights on or being abused. It's time for people on this planet to thrive.

We need to feed our creativity and recognize the faulty, limited beliefs we're telling ourselves that keep us stuck. Don't sort through your past like belongings in the attic. Now is not the time to decide what you want to get rid of and what you want to keep. It's time to be aware of your ability to craft a new world. We still have our story but now we should think of it in parable form, not as facts. It was just a story we told ourselves to learn lessons. We should be like my niece and start creating a new story of abundance, generosity and peace of soul. We have a lot invested in our past. But do we want to invest more in something we don't need? If you came into some money would you invest in 8-track players? This invention only exists as memorabilia. It's a marker in time not an ingredient for your future. Discussing the past can create feelings of nostalgia and occasionally stress. Our memories deserve periodic reflection if they can move us immediately forward.

Staying connected to a divine flow is a challenge. Certainly, there will be times of emotional upheaval but it is vital you regain your strength of spirit as quickly as possible. A body that is mentally, physically and spiritually nourished will guide you towards the life you desire. While you prepare healthy food in the morning, listen to a podcast or watch a video on manifesting the life of your dreams. I used to teach a goal-setting workshop. Initially, we would focus on these three words: Be, Do, Have. Many people believe in order to **be** the person they want to be, they have to **have** something. With this limited belief, you may not ever take the action necessary to attain your goals. However, if you start with *being* the person you want to be, and then *doing* things in accordance with this being, you stand a better chance at *having* what you are seeking. The trap is when *having* a possession represents your identity. Be clear about what it is you want to have. Make sure if what you seek is a possession it doesn't determine who you are. If what you seek is happiness and you believe a person or a material object will bring it, you're still trapped. What is it you want to have and why?

If I am what I have and I lose what I have, who then am I?
Erich Fromm

You have to clear your thoughts of self-limiting beliefs. Just as cleansing your body is absolutely necessary for thriving, you will need to cleanse your mind for true happiness and fulfillment. Running water clears itself. Stagnant water is a breeding ground for disease. A mind free from stagnation is a mind cleared for creation. It's as important to keep your life flowing forward and to clear stagnant thoughts, as it is to drink pure clean water. We think about 60,000 thoughts a day. How many of yours are positive and make you feel good about yourself? How many thoughts inspire you to live the life of your dreams? There is a Zen saying: *A cup that is full hath no room for more.* In other words, if you think you already have all of the answers, your cup will be full. If you're experiencing stress in your life, maybe it's time to empty your cup and allow a new awareness to fill your presence.

The life of strain is difficult. The life of inner peace, being harmonious and without stress, is the easiest type of existence.
Norman Vincent Peale *The Power of Positive Thinking*

By examining your biological processes more intricately, you can see how your ability to feel true peace can be disrupted on a subtle level 24 hours a day. Taking the time to understand these processes, will give you greater control over your health and satisfaction in life. By cultivating peace in your mind and body you can live a life of ease in harmony with your environment.

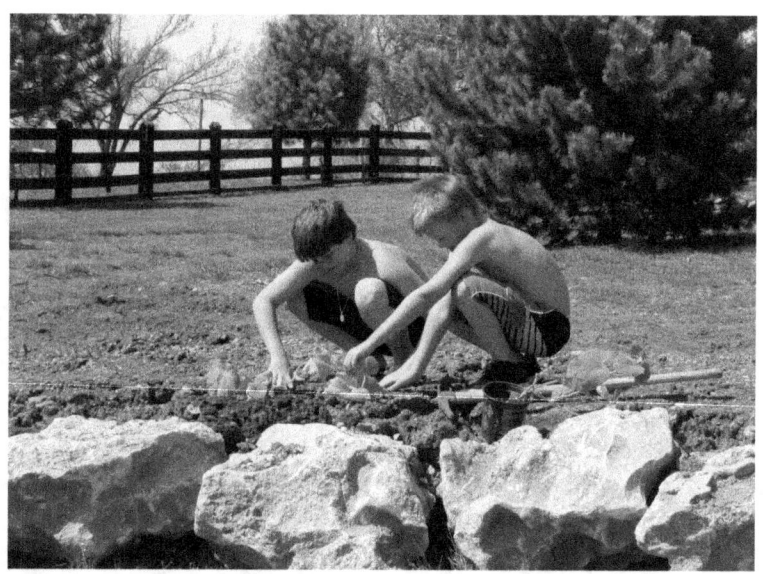

If you think in terms of a year, plant a seed; if in terms of ten years, plant trees; if in terms of 100 years, teach the people.

Confucius

CHAPTER 12

SURTHRIVAL OF THE FITTEST

*Though the problems of the world are increasingly complex,
the solutions remain embarrassingly simple.*
Bill Mollison Father of Permaculture

In order to affect real change in the world, we will most likely need to simplify our lives. The resources of this planet are limited. The landfills are growing exponentially and pollution, whether or not it is a factor in climate change is not ignorable. Most of our water is contaminated and disease is on the rise. According to *The Healthy Farmland Diet:* "Only about 2 percent of U.S. cropland is used to grow fruits and vegetables, while 59 percent is devoted to commodity crops, such as corn and soybeans, which are used primarily to produce three things: meat, processed foods such as high fructose corn syrup, and biofuels such as ethanol."[1] Permaculture aims to help heal the land and even addresses our economics so we can make the transition from being dependent consumers to becoming responsible producers.[2] The ethics of permaculture are: *People Care, Earth Care, Fair Share.* Jacque Fresco, futurist, organized *The Venus Project.* Fresco's life's work has been dedicated to redesigning our communities based on, but not limited to, social cooperation and natural resource management. *The Venus Project* promotes environmentally friendly, humane lifestyles and seeks to eliminate elitism while addressing our current dehumanizing monetary system.[3]

We have tremendous opportunities available to us but it will take a collective effort to create a new reality. Unfortunately, even though we're members of a community, we spend vast amounts of time separated in our homes, cars and offices, feeling isolation instead of connection. Consider forming a *Meetup* group in your area for people interested in reaching their potential, caring for the land or sharing goods and services. Many times, people agree with me about being self-reliant then follow it with the fact that they're too busy. Other times, people say they don't enjoy things like gardening. That's understandable. I don't enjoy mowing my lawn. This is where I think it would be beneficial to barter for goods and services locally. Instead of tractor trailers hauling things across the country or barges occasionally spilling their contents into the ocean, we could take an inventory of what we really need and encourage the local community to rise to the occasion of self-reliance and sustainability. If we started the conversation of barter in our communities, we may find there is a wealth of talented individuals longing for the chance to provide something we need. Even creating a community garden will get people talking about important issues surrounding health and the environment, not to mention all of the wonderful food you'll grow.

When I first began to make radical changes in my life, I went through my house and took a mental inventory of the things I needed. Notice I didn't say things I *couldn't live without*. My home contains many things that in reality I don't need. The confusing part is that I spent what could have been *free time* earning money to acquire useless possessions, some of which are destined for the landfill. Unfortunately, we often rely on material items to give us a sense of self-worth and allow possessions to affect our opinions of others. We respect people for what they own instead of who they are. It's no wonder so many people are unhappy. It's easier to disconnect from consumerism when you see through the illusion of material happiness. Once I reduced my need for possessions, I was able to work less and enjoy more freedom. I took another inventory of the food in my home. I wanted to find out what percentage of it had an origin I could trust. I was curious to see how much of it contained empty calories, harmful toxic dyes, chemicals and high fructose corn syrup. Every time I went to the store, I committed to buying more environmentally responsible, nutritious food.

We have more control over our lives than we realize. Many people are stuck in limited belief patterns about their own potential for health and happiness. They blame their *genes*, their *metabolism*, and their *past*. Know that your genes are not the end of the road. You can affect *genes* through your food choices. Even more amazing is that you can affect your genes through awareness. In the book, *The Biology of Belief,* Bruce Lipton, a geneticist, explains how our state of mind can improve our genetic function.[4] All *metabolism* is enzyme based. We are born with a bank account of enzymes and it begins to decline in our 30's. Our bodies are capable of creating enzymes when fed on proper nutrition. Consuming quality living food and taking supplemental enzymes will improve your metabolism. Our *pasts* or beliefs about who we are and what we're capable of are based on vast amounts of misinformation. Read *The Untethered Soul* by Michael Singer to more fully free your mind from your past.

Once you realize you have the power to make radical change in your life, you can become truly happy, healthy and self-reliant. With proper cleansing and regeneration of our minds and bodies, we become clearer. It's easier to see the ultimate truths of brotherhood, spirit and the connection to Earth as a living entity when you are focused on thriving. Self-love is regenerated through proper care of ourselves, service to others and by being responsible stewards of the planet. As more people tune into their human potential, a critical mass of prospering will ensue. I can think of nothing nobler than a collective effort to create a better world for future generations.

In 2011, the town where I live was ripped apart by an F5 tornado. The resolve and commitment by our community to help one another that dreadful night and the months to follow was astonishing. Despite the devastation, we demonstrated solidarity and union that struck the hearts of the nation. People from around the globe offered their love and labor. Even though we were in pain, we felt oneness and hope. Now that we have nearly restored our city, the memories of that fateful night are beginning to fade. We have returned to our homes and isolation. I wonder sometimes if the residents here miss those months when we were all unified in a life of meaning and constant service to others. We may be content but deep down inside we know we're capable of more. We lived it.

Human beings have the capacity to actualize amazing possibilities. I believe strongly that if we commanded control of our bodies and minds, we would resist the political control imposed upon us. At the time of this writing, our country is considering the task of providing national health care. For a moment, consider an alternate future. Imagine every individual reevaluating their health and upgrading all of their choices. What if we stopped purchasing food from factory monoculture farms that are inhumane and contributing to widespread pollution and contamination? What if every single person supported local sustainable farms or grew their food, learned about Mother Nature's medicine and consumed high-quality water? What if everyone recognized their power, meditated on self-love and felt the healing effects of a positive attitude? Without an insatiable need to spend and consume, we could work less. We could focus on self-mastery instead of materialism. Daily, people could spend time outdoors, enjoying their families, community, sunshine and grounding. We could put our bodies to full use with healthy activities and develop deeper levels of consciousness, unlocking the power of our minds. We could all improve our athletic and musical ability.

With these simple steps, we could vote with every dollar we spend to reduce corrupt corporations funding the campaigns of corrupt politicians. We could improve our immune function and have fewer visits to the doctor. Life threatening, chronic illnesses would diminish. With more freedom and fewer illnesses we might effectively manage stress, resulting in decreased rates of smoking. With fewer episodes of depression, poor health and lack of self-love, alcohol consumption would also decrease. If we all simplified our lives, upgraded our nutrition and assumed more responsibility for our health, national health care may not even be an issue.

Currently, we have choices when it comes to the care of our bodies, but if we continue to give others control over our health, one day we may find many of our choices have been eliminated. By making a tremendous effort to care for my body, I don't find myself in the doctor's office and I haven't taken a prescription in many years. Apart from the occurrence of a natural disaster or other accident, I feel with proper care, I can continue to avoid serious illnesses. Therefore, I don't wish to be a part of a national health care plan and I certainly don't want to be penalized for not joining a system I have no intention of using. Personally, I spend a fair amount of my discretionary income upgrading my nutrition and taking preventive measures to avoid illness. Even though I don't buy subsidized food, my tax dollars still go into the pockets of the corporations producing it. I'd prefer to limit the amount of money I pay for government programs I don't condone. Since everyone has different opinions about the programs we support and the ones we don't, it seems that limiting government programs in general would reduce our differences.

I'm very passionate when it comes to the topic of national health care for when decisions get made at the federal level, making changes at the state level becomes nearly impossible. I believe the more responsibility we give to the government, the less responsible we will be. Furthermore, our current health care system revolves around pharmaceuticals and I believe this is contributing to many unintended consequences. According to David Alan Goodman Ph.D., neuroscientist at Newport Neuroscience Center, almost all drugs (approved and illicit) cause damage to the prefrontal cortex when taken long-term, preventing you from accessing higher nervous system activity while diminishing human prefrontal lobe abilities.[5] The ramifications of this information were profound to me. After corresponding with Dr. Goodman, it became imminently clear that living a drug-free lifestyle would contribute to my ability to experience higher brain function.

Recently, people were discussing a vaccine for shingles that costs over $200. They mentioned the vaccine is only 70% effective but if you do get shingles after having had the vaccine, your symptoms wouldn't be as severe. This statement seemed to lack verisimilitude. Being only 70% effective was not reassuring. Furthermore, it seemed there would be no scientific way to study the statement about symptoms. How can you **prove** your symptoms of a disease *you didn't get* would be less severe if you got it for the first time? Even if there were some science to support the claim, I would not be influenced to get the shot because I avoid medications at all costs. I've only had one vaccination in my life and that was because I couldn't attend university without it. Personally, I worry that if national health care goes into affect, I will be forced to get more vaccinations. If I had an allergy to eggs, I wouldn't have to get the shots but I'm not allergic to eggs. However, I am allergic to the versions of the diseases vaccines contain and other typical vaccine ingredients such as formaldehyde, aluminum, mercury, GMO's, crossbred bacteria from animals, mosquitoes, and diseased humans, as well as hormones from infected cows, pigs, chickens and monkeys.[6]

People already repeat the propaganda that by my not getting a vaccine, I'll make everyone else sick. My reply is always the same, "If your vaccines worked, I would pose no risk for you." I'm hoping they'll conclude that their vaccines aren't working as well as their own immune systems would if they gave their bodies what they truly needed to prevent disease. Instead of concluding that vaccines potentially do more harm than good, people usually end up saying something about polio. This is the standard defense and again, I find it to be a frustrating reply. This disease was already on the decline prior to the vaccination due to clean water and improved sanitation.[7] Additionally, if the polio vaccine is so effective why can't this disease be eradicated in India, the Congo and underdeveloped countries?

Being discerning when it came to scientific studies was of prime importance while returning my body to health. You can get statistics to tell you anything you want if you torture the numbers long enough.[8] With any research, I tried to find out who funded the study and asked *cui bono?* Following the money and finding out who benefited from the findings of the study, helped me to make more informed decisions. If a pharmaceutical company provided the data, I wondered, are these numbers honestly serving humanity or their shareholders? Phil Angell from Monsanto, a company in the genetically modified food industry, told a writer for New York Times Magazine, "Monsanto should not have to vouchsafe the safety of biotech food. Our interest is in selling as much of it as possible. Assuring its safety is the F.D.A.'s job."[9] The problem is that somewhere along the line, the safety of these foods falls into the twilight zone. The toxins in GMO food are not the F.D.A.'s responsibility; they are under the jurisdiction of the E.P.A. The health of the food and the toxins combined seems to be overlooked; therefore, many consumers remain unaware of their harm. Looking deeper into the regulatory system allowed me to see that this was not an unintentional oversight.

In a world where people were telling me what to think, I found that learning a solid process of reasoning was instrumental to having a healthy mind. In order to make better decisions about my health, I became aware of logical fallacies. Through online educational videos, I learned to listen for these fallacies to improve my critical thinking skills. To enhance my ability to reason, I needed to improve my brain's ability to function. If minerals essentially run my cells, then how well were my brain cells functioning if my food choices were starkly deficient in minerals? By relying on substandard sources for my nutrition, my brain would pay the price and my perspective would suffer the cost. By improving my sources for information, I was able to make more informed decisions.

Today, government interference and compulsory schooling has diminished our creative thinking skills and individual problem solving is on the decline. Our education system is based on the Prussian model of social obedience and the indoctrination that the King is always right.[10] After reading through a book online involving the U. S. Department of Education called *The Deliberate Dumbing Down of America,* I began to question what was happening in our schools.[11] The increase in standardized testing and the controls imposed on teachers to improve scores is disconcerting. The freedom and creativity of children is being systematically removed through the acclimation of more rules. Consequently, children indoctrinated into a system of control will be more accepting of a *nanny state* and this is unfortunate because they are our future.

At most public schools, poor quality food and the lack of freedom to time meals appropriately, contribute to stress in the bodies and minds of children, resulting in poor behavior. One day, I went to my nephew's school to join him for lunch. Afterwards, I saw his class was outside running laps before I even left the parking lot. It bothered me because I knew the blood flow needed to be in the core for at least an hour after eating for proper digestion. If the kids go running right after a meal, their blood will flow to their extremities preventing proper digestion, nutrient delivery and ultimately, peace of mind. Even subtle stress in the body will contribute to behavior problems. Consequently, regular disciplinary actions lead to a lack of self-worth and an increase in medications to manage disruptions.

I have a high regard and immense respect for teachers. I feel it's the federal system that is constricting the students and the teachers alike. If the federal government had less of a role in education, I believe there would be a surge in creativity and self-worth. With greater freedom, I believe children would discover their true passions. Sadly, children are led to believe their best chance at happiness is through higher education and more money.

In this day and age, despite our higher education and scientific discoveries, poor health is on the rise and personal responsibility for our health is on the decline. Medical intervention is increasing and holistic self-care is decreasing. If we are to truly heal, we must assume responsibility for our own health. Rather than demanding access to insurance and physicians, we should devise a plan for higher quality food, pure water and air that is not polluted. Instead of assuming someone else will purify these basic needs, we should consider our role in their contamination. By examining the consequences of our actions, we can reduce pollution of the land and improve our chances for health.

> *Optimism is a strategy for making a better future.*
> *Because unless you believe that the future can be better,*
> *you are unlikely to step up and take responsibility for making it so.*
> Noam Chomsky

When you have a clear picture of the toxins in our world, you not only recognize the importance of holistic nutrition, you accept the idea of cleansing. The immune system cannot function at its peak when it's constantly exposed to toxins. Like a country, peace isn't possible until the war has stopped. Rebuilding isn't an option when a country is still under attack. A body won't heal until the war has ended. To our dismay, we live in a world of increasing toxicity; therefore, cleansing needs to be a consistent part of one's life. We are ultimately responsible for our health.

There isn't an insurance program for this way of life so one must be diligent. Natural medicine isn't part of the national plan due to a lack of scientific support for self-healing. Many health care professionals have admitted they only had a few hours of nutrition education. For this reason, some doctors and nurses know very little about holistic lifestyles. You won't find subjects in medical research who are reaching their genetic potential for health. People who heal themselves fall into the category of placebo during pharmaceutical studies and their results are discarded. They are considered to be anomalies and are of no use in proving the effectiveness of drugs. Usually subjects who are susceptible to placebo are identified and removed before the study begins. Imagine how different medicine would be if more resources were devoted to studying self-healing or *the placebo effect.*

The law of floatation was not discovered by contemplating
the sinking of things, but by contemplating things which
floated naturally and then intelligently asking why they did so.
Thomas Troward

If we simplified our lives, the complex dysfunction in our bodies would diminish. If we respected trade schools and autodidactic methods of learning as much as we respected higher education, we would see an increase in self-worth and entrepreneurship. By reducing corporatism and restoring local family businesses, we could improve the health of our communities. With fewer people in factories and more people devoted to conscientious food production, the health of the nation would improve. Sadly, many people are more concerned with what they are putting on their bodies instead of what they are putting in them. The amount of energy and resources spent trying to feel good about ourselves through materialism and status, could be invested in improving our health, talents and wisdom. With a solid sense of self and improved responses to life, we wouldn't be so easily shaken by the opinions of others and one's prudential value would be higher. If self-reliance became a top priority in our communities, we would exponentially increase our chances of reaching our human potential.

When you finally find there is no way out but self-awareness
and the incredible pain and loneliness and responsibility it
brings, then and only then will you begin to be alive,
and begin to know the joy of freedom.
Paul Williams *Das Energi*

If you want happiness for a lifetime, help the next generation.
Chinese Proverb

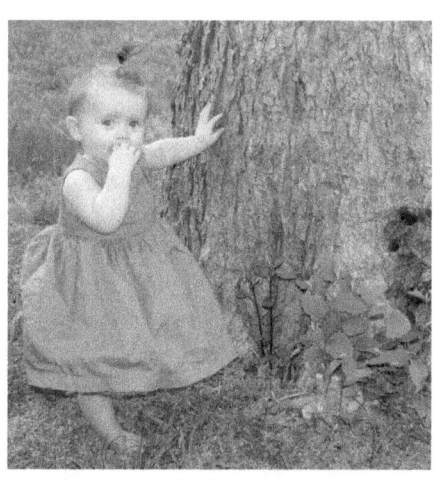

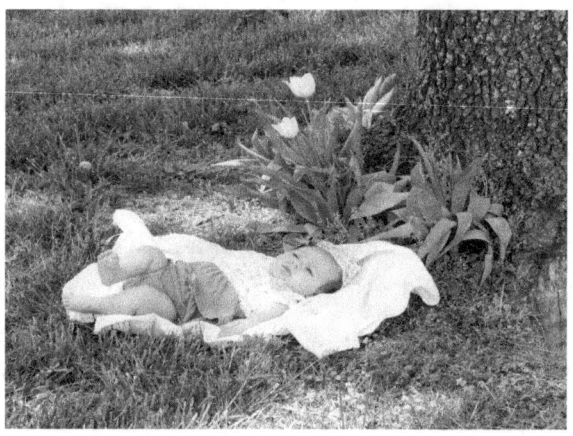

I believe that to meet the challenge of our times, human beings will have to develop a greater sense of universal responsibility. We must all learn to work not just for our own self, family, or nation but for the benefit of all humankind. Universal responsibility is the key to human survival. It is the best foundation for world peace, the equitable use of natural resources, and through concern for future generations, the proper care of the environment.
The Dalai Lama

CHAPTER 13

BEAUTY AND THE BEAST

No problem can be solved from the same
level of consciousness that created it.
Albert Einstein

When I used to see people struggling, I would search my transcendental treasure chest for the right words to help restore peace of mind. However, the older I get, I see it will take more earthly treasures to create harmony. Even though many of our problems are conceptual in nature, their origins can be quite physical. The brain guides the body in the same way the subconscious shapes the consciousness. Similarly, the brain is at the mercy of the body, just as the subconscious mind is at the mercy of one's conscious attention.

When the body begins to experience stress, the mind follows suit. It's subtle. Rarely will you feel the shift. Even subtle stress in the brain can activate fight, flight or freeze, influencing your reactions and your view of life. When you function from the regions of the brain responsible for higher consciousness, you are able to process information more effectively and responsibly. When I become discouraged and only see problems around me, I sit back for a moment and consider my nutrition over the last 24 hours. It's a simple solution but sometimes all it takes to shift my mind into peace is awareness that

I'm operating from survival due to poor nutrition. This clouds my view of the world and when I apply the law of attraction to this state, more stress will follow.

It's easy to attribute external factors to your stress, giving yourself reasons for unhappiness or excuses for suffering. However, if you were able to hear the cries of your cells, longing for pure water and minerals, you might more clearly understand why your view of the world has begun to shift from hope to despair. In order to create solutions for happiness, one needs to be experiencing peace in the body and mind. When my body is at peace, my view is one of optimism not dissatisfaction.

After restoring harmony in the body, the alarms in the mind become quiet and one can approach life with greater clarity. In order to live the life of my dreams, I need a brain that isn't in survival mode. This requires a consistent effort to be present and cultivate moment-to-moment awareness of the world in which I live. Even though I can name outside reasons for the problems in my life, it doesn't mean my views are accurate. There are so many factors at play for any given situation that true understanding is overwhelming. Instead of spending too much time on the past, I have gratitude for my life and put efforts towards a sustainable future. My awareness truly expanded when I improved my actions involving the environment that sustains life.

When my cells were not getting the necessary minerals to improve enzymatic reactions and protein function, my body was not in harmony. Before I made radical change, I was regularly exposing my body to toxins. The energy required for cleansing these harmful elements was utilizing energy that could've been used to reach peak states of happiness. When my cells had to protect themselves from pollutants they weren't in a state of growth. If my cells weren't in a state of growth, how could I honestly say that I was growing as a person? When I took the time to examine my thoughts throughout the day, I was able to see which ones were centered in growth verses protection.

Can you differentiate which of your reactions and thoughts are centered in growth and which ones stem from protection? Fight, flight and freeze are protection systems. It's easy to examine momentous scenarios and label your reactions. Potentially, subtle stress has caused you to have a less dramatic response to life, making it harder to recognize survival modes. Recreate your last stressful morning and see if you can recognize which protection response was activated. Then imagine how you would have handled your adversities if you were in a state of growth. If I'm responding to scenarios with behaviors that conflict with loving, kind awareness, I'm in stress. If I cultivate a compassionate, loving mind, my chances of returning to a state of harmony are even greater.

Sometimes the lack of energy from poor food contributes to an inability to alter your course. When your worldview is shaped by subtle or possibly dire stress in your physical body, all you may see are problems without solutions. On the contrary, think of being in love. It has the power to completely overrule your perspective. When feeling love, you don't notice the same amount of dissatisfaction. There's no desire for complaining when you are consumed with desire for your loved one. Even though nothing in your external world has changed, your view is suddenly pleasant. The healing power of love can override poor nutritional choices. If you're not in love, being positive and forgiving towards yourself when you slip from peak nutrition will be instrumental in reducing stress. Even though positive emotions surrounding your food have the ability to override potential ill-effects, they can't indefinitely be substituted for high quality food and water. Occasionally, you can be gentle with yourself if you waver but if you waver more often than not, positive thinking may not prove to be beneficial. As a matter of fact, as you are potentially starting to see, positive thinking may not be possible if you can't take your body out of stress.

Even people in love need to eat eventually. If they want their relationships and their bodies to be healthy long term, they will need to make high quality choices when it comes to nutrition. Unfortunately, blissful feelings of love fade over time. This is why mini-meditations on self-love throughout the day will help keep feelings of love alive. Self-reliance in this area will prevent feelings of dependency. Consequently, if you're not relying on another to feel peace, you may not blame someone if you're feeling sadness. If you're not practicing this awareness and your nutrition is suffering, a cascade of problems may unfold before you. By not managing your blood sugar effectively, dopamine will be low and you might turn to addictive behaviors to reach peak states of reward and pleasure when true love and health are lacking. I believe improving these areas of our lives will lead to decreased: infidelity, alcoholism, gambling, drug addiction and destruction of the family unit.

If you are feeling self-love, keeping your body out of stress and improving your peace of mind, you might find that you reach new levels of consciousness in your relationships. You may discover the idea of finding a new love interest pales in comparison to creating a conscientious, healthy, loving, extraordinary bond with your current partner. If you're single and looking to unite with another, elevate your expectations to a new level of interacting. If more people become aware of their potential, the opportunities to meet conscientious, healthy, loving people will increase exponentially. With people fulfilling their need for love and achieving mastery over their bodies and minds, hopefully, consumerism and destruction of the planet will finally wane.

It's profound when you realize how linked your nutrition is to your worldview. It strongly influences how you will respond to life and can be empowering when you see the amount of control you actually have over your satisfaction. Recognizing you have a choice to shift your mind from survival to happiness is key. It's imperative that you take deep breaths before you react to emotional stress to access a more conscientious state. If someone is treating you poorly, take a moment to realize that possibly their body is in stress and they're not reacting from their higher place of consciousness. Just because you're interacting with someone who is in stress, doesn't mean you have to believe you're responsible for it, regardless if they're blaming you or not. With a balanced mind and body you can come up with solutions instead of blame.

I believe a good portion of our creativity manifests out of stress and insecurity. At times in my life when I'm facing big problems, I can be very creative about how I'll remedy the situation. My need for survival causes me to generate ideas and plans for how I'll overcome the challenges I'm facing. If the solutions I devise are noble and involve helping others, I know I've tapped into the positive energy of creation. If my goals are namely self-serving, disguised as service to others, I know I'm still motivated by survival. In this mode, I continue to feel my needs are not being met and I need to have more than or be better than others in order to abolish any chance of failure or defeat. This will ultimately lead to more stress and less satisfaction in life. Consequently, my accomplishments will never be enough if I'm in a state of protection and my acquisitions will never fill the void. The lives I touch may not truly benefit from my presence if I'm trapped in the illusion of surviving instead of thriving.

Striving to be better than others is not to be confused with self-mastery. Mastery over your body and mind is admirable; mastery over others is not. We should aspire to reach our full potential and elevate others with what we've learned. I feel honored when a great teacher freely shares knowledge because they're excited to share the experience of growth. When sharing information, tune into higher consciousness, otherwise, true knowledge can be lost and the ego found. We should all hope for our fellow man to feel self-worth and be abundantly sustained and fulfilled.

Our bodies mirror our world. Sometimes when I see people fighting and competing, I think of the human body fighting within itself to overcome a disease. When our nutrition is inadequate, our cells will compete for minerals. If a person gets an infection he may take an antibiotic that wipes out good and bad bacteria because the medicine can't differentiate. When a country goes to war, the casualties of war also extend beyond the people considered to be bad. If we increase the number of beneficial bacteria in our bodies, the harmful bacteria do not cause illness. We have potentially harmful bacteria in our bodies all of the time. However, through the overuse of antibiotics, good bacteria are on the decline. If we increase the number of healthy people in our cities, national health care becomes less of a burden. Unfortunately, the number of unhealthy people in our world is on the rise. It comes as no surprise that unhealthy people will ask for medicine and an unhealthy country will demand a war.

When I see the *world that has been pulled over our eyes,*[1] I have to wonder how much of it was created out of stress? How many of our corporations contribute to the greater good of humanity? There is an elaborate system of controls we impose upon ourselves in order to belong, hopefully find a mate, to respect ourselves according to society's superficial standards. Yet if the machine was created out of insecurity and fear, how much more of ourselves do we want to give it? I don't want to work until I'm too feeble to enjoy retirement because my body has deteriorated due to the ill-effects of poor nutrition, pollution, materialism and greed.

Daily, people disregard the unfair distribution of wealth. Potentially, this lack of concern continues because some people believe the poor and impoverished should save themselves. If you've ever felt powerless to change the world, imagine how the poor feel. Surviving on cheap subsidized food; their bodies are surely in stress and their hope diminished. Neighborhood and community gardens for the poor and homeless would be beautiful projects. I've heard elitists say you can't feed the poor because they will continue to have children and the problems will only get worse. Again, I suggest we approach it from another angle. Stop feeding the beast of materialism, elitism and greed and see what happens.

Clearly, the world is facing big challenges. Fortunately, you have the power to make a difference in your life. Restore harmony in your body, reach peace in your mind and detach from exterior self-worth. Inspire children to be environmentally responsible and autonomous. Reach out in your community to create a network of support. Vote with your dollars to support sustainability and conscientious companies. Love yourself, have compassion for others and imagine the possibilities of self-mastery.

There is an Arabic saying: *Don't wake a slave; he may be dreaming that he is free.* Bhagwan Shree Rajneesh says in *The Book of Wisdom II* that whenever awakening happens, people become antagonistic. He postulates, "The world is fast asleep and people are enjoying their dreams." They are decorating their dreams and making them comfortable. If someone suggests they're sleeping, the sleepers are offended because once they wake and the dream is gone, they feel they will be left with suffering and nothing else. They're not yet aware of the great peace to be found beyond their misery.[2] When we open our eyes to all of the promise and beauty that surrounds us, our minds will mirror our potential for mastery and true freedom.

Sometimes it falls upon a generation to be great.
You can be that great generation.
Nelson Mandela

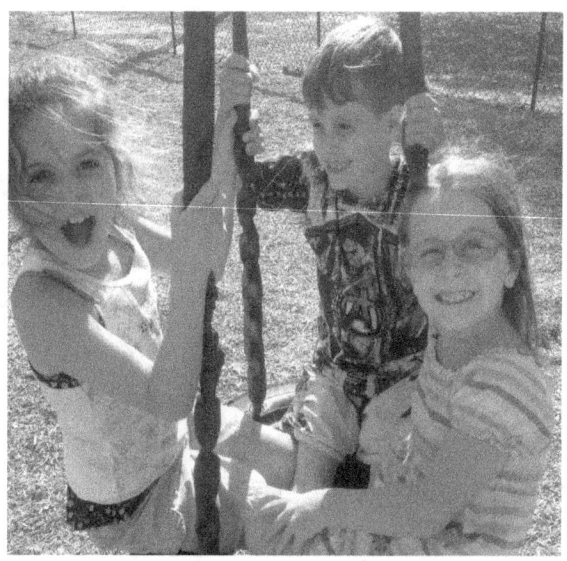

The Beginning...

APPENDIX I

The following questions are for your consideration or to be discussed with others.

If the companies with F ratings fail, what kinds of jobs could we create to sustain life on this planet, responsibly?

If the top priority of our community became conscientious, local food production, we could return land to biodiversity and sustainable farming. Imagine all of the jobs we would need in order to provide our community's food supply.

On your next drive down a busy street, look at the companies you see. How would these businesses need to change in order to support a more responsible existence? Which ones would disappear in a culture of awakened consciousness?

If more giant corporations failed, we would need more entrepreneurs. What would you want to do in order to support yourself or your family? Would you want to become an artisan or a teacher? If you became an artisan, what would you like to create? What would you teach?

If parents saved for their child's entrepreneurship instead of college, financial worries may not even be an issue once adulthood is reached. Through trade schools and apprenticeships, passions could form into lasting, satisfying careers. What kind of plan could you devise for your child's future in lieu of a college career?

In an ideal world, whom would you become to contribute to sustainable life on this planet?

Imagine you have reached peak fitness and your goal weight. What kind of lifestyle would you live to care for yourself? What kinds of things would you stop doing today that normally you might allow?

Is your emotional pain real? If your thoughts are painful and you stop paying attention to your thoughts, is the problem still there? If a tree falls in the woods and no one is there to hear it, does it still make a sound? I don't know, but I do know if you aren't there in the woods, you won't hear it. In the same regard if you are not listening to the voice in your head, you won't hear it. If the voice in your head is filled with sad ideas and you return to clear, quiet presence, you will not feel the pain of your thoughts.

Is being alone painful or is it the thought of being alone? If you reached your genetic potential, would you know the interconnectedness of all life? Would you still feel alone if you knew all of life is connected? Are the reasons why you are alone still painful if they are based on misinformation?

If you jailed a person for a crime they didn't commit, would you keep them imprisoned even after you learned the truth of their innocence? Who is it inside of you that is imprisoned for false beliefs? Outside of yourself, whom are you still punishing for crimes they committed out of misinformation? Possibly, it's someone you need to love and release from the confines of the prison in your mind.

If your opinion of me were based on misinformation, why would I allow myself to be hurt by your opinions? How many times have we allowed the opinions of others to dictate how we feel about ourselves?

If you couldn't turn to the doctor for every ailment, what would you do?

What's stopping you from taking full responsibility for your life now?

When you're faced with death, you begin to question what is really important in life. Ask yourself what your top priorities would be if you could only live a few more days. What's preventing you from living in accordance with your top priorities now?

If there were a collapse of our current world, would you be able to survive?

According to the creators of the documentary *Consumed: Inside the Belly of the Beast*, "Transition Towns, recycling, alternative power, and enduring design, are just attacking the symptoms. They are merely allowing us to continue living the way we are. They are buying us time, not embracing the root cause, our psychology."[1] Do you think our psychology is contributing to the extinction of our species?

There are no passengers on Spaceship Earth. We are all crew.
Marshall McLuhan

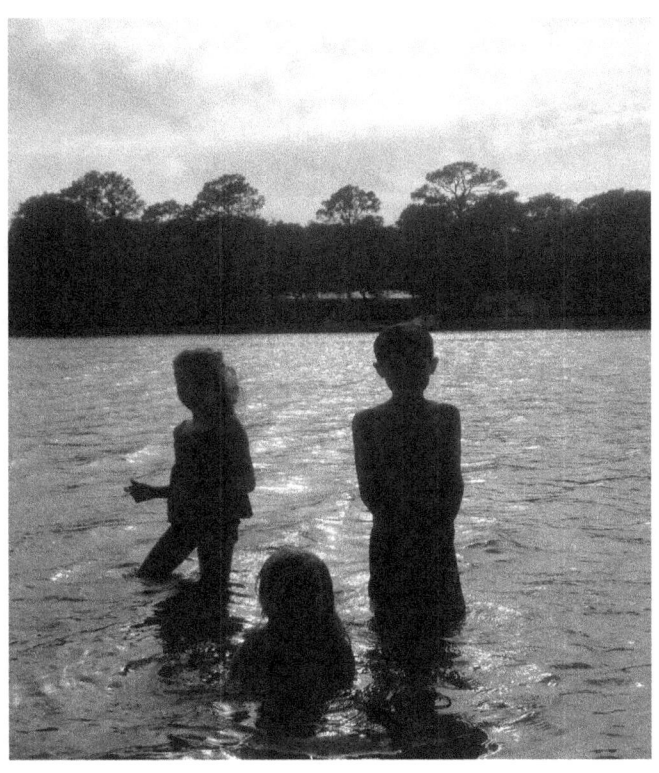

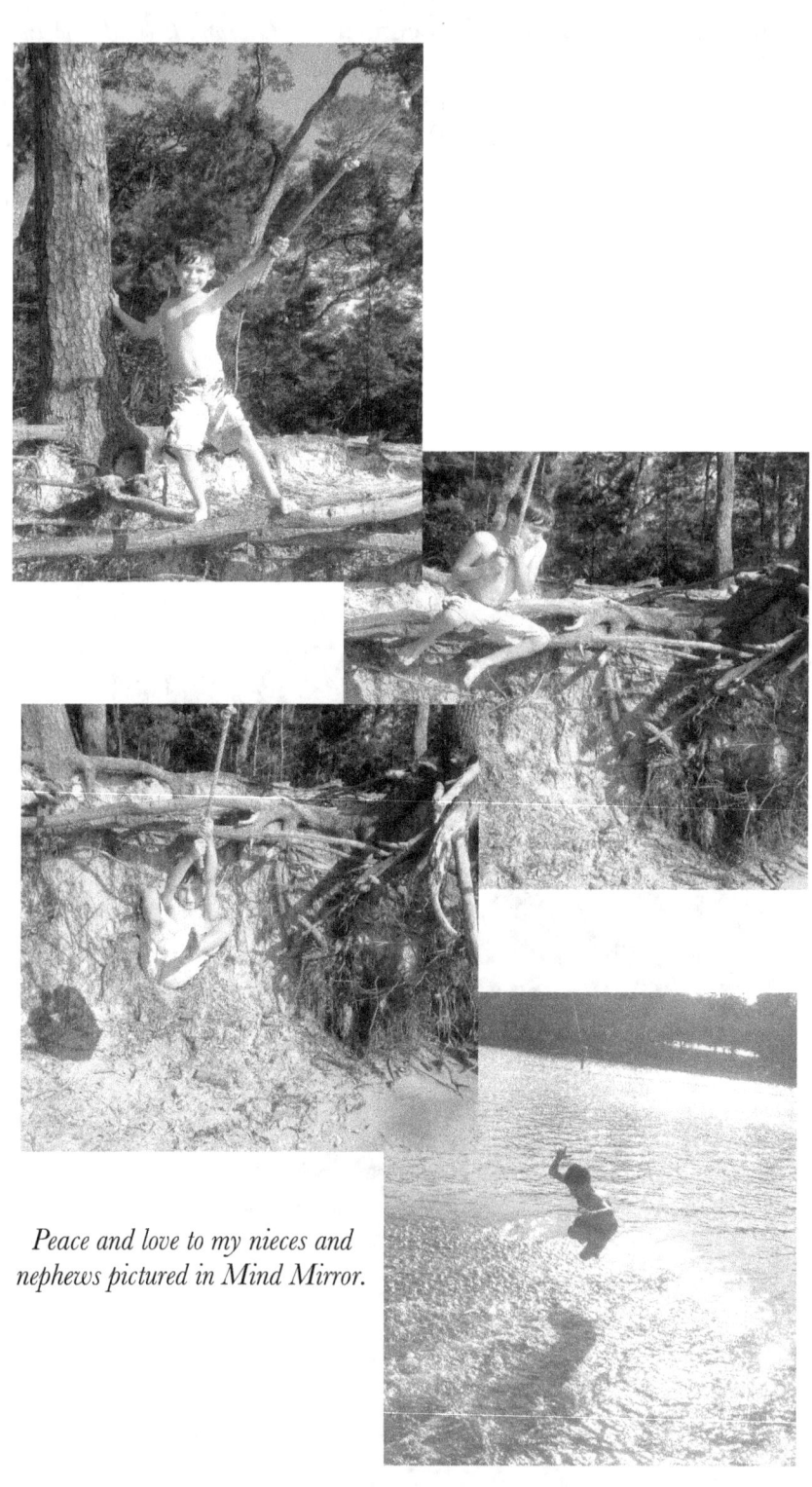

Peace and love to my nieces and nephews pictured in Mind Mirror.

APPENDIX II

Visit: http://www.mindmirror.org for resource videos and links to support the material. To schedule Christa for public speaking, workshops or video chat at your book club meeting, email her through the website.

Recommended Documentaries Streaming on Netflix:
I Am
Food, Inc.
Hungry for Change
Food Matters
Future of Food
Fresh
Fat Sick and Nearly Dead

Documentaries On YouTube:
Consumed: Inside the Belly of the Beast
Consuming Kids: The Commercialization of Children
State of Mind: Psychology of Control
The Ultimate History Lesson

Food supplement suppliers:
http://www.longevitywarehouse.com
http://www.traceminerals.com
http://www.surthrival.com
http://www.naturalnews.com
http://www.mountainroseherbs.com
http://www.ultimatesuperfoods.com
http://www.upgradedself.com

Podcasts: Patrick Timpone's interviews with David Wolfe, Daniel Vitalis, Mike Adams and many more experts in the field of nutrition and awakening to your potential can be found at: www.oneradionetwork.com.

Gastric Empty Times (digestion) : Approximations**
Morning drink : 5 minutes
Piece of fruit : 15 - 30 minutes
Fruit/vegetable juice or broths : 15 - 30 minutes
Smoothies : 30 minutes - 1 hour
Vegetables, Eggs, or Fish : 1 hour
Grains & Beans : 1.5 - 2 hours
Seeds, Nuts : 2 - 3 hours
Dairy : 2 - 5 hours (Skim and low fat options : 90 minutes)
Meat : 2 - 5 hours (Chicken is on the low end and pork is on the high end of this time.)
Typical meal on average : 1.5 - 3 hours

**Digestion times vary according to the health of the individual, food combinations, proper chewing of food and the addition of foreign chemicals and dyes.

To better understand meal timing for improving insulin resistance, you could hire a BodyMind Nutritionist. To become a BodyMind Nutritionist visit: http://www.bodymindinstitute.com

My version of the morning drink:
8-10 oz living water
½ cup of organic juice
10 Drops of ConcenTrace®
1/4 tsp high quality salt
1 ml Ionic Magnesium**
.5 tsp TMG***
Nascent Iodine

** Magnesium is severely lacking in our food and the majority of the population is deficient. This wonderful mineral has a positive effect on numerous conditions from appetite to blood pressure regulation.

*** David Wolfe discusses TMG for hormone balancing and detoxification during interviews on One Radio Network.

NOTES

PART I

Chapter 2

1. Jones, Elliot, *Better World Shopping Guide: Every Dollar Makes a Difference*
http://www.betterworldshopper.org
The application for your mobile device is called *Better World Shopper*

PART II

Chapter 3

1. Ruiz, Don Miguel, *The Voice of Knowledge* (2004) p. 83
2. Gazzaniga, Michael, *The Ethical Brain* (2005) Location 1835 (Kindle edition)
3. Gladwell, Malcolm, *Blink: The Power of Thinking Without Thinking* (2005)
To experience examples of your unconscious behavior search for AIT Tests by Malcolm Gladwell or follow this link:
https://implicit.harvard.edu/implicit/user/agg/blindspot/tablet.htm
4. Taylor, John Maxwell, *The Power of I Am: Creating a New World of Enlightened Personal Interaction,* (2006) pp. 10-12
5. Prather, Hugh, *Notes to Myself: My Struggle to Become a Person* (1983) p. 91

Chapter 4

1. David Wolfe interview on the importance of salt: (2011)
http://www.youtube.com/watch?v=3XJCnanT4ac

2. Rodale News article on chemicals in plastic by Emily Main (2011)
http://www.rodalenews.com/chemicals-plastic

3. www.berkeyfilters.com

4. Fluoride:

www.fluoridealert.org   www.fluoridedebate.com

5. http://www.naturalnews.com/030952_CDC_fluoride.html

6. Information presented during *The 90 Day BodyMind Renewal Program* at The BodyMind Institute by Lars Gustafsson http://www.bodymindinstitute.com

7. Emoto, Masaru, *The Hidden Messages in Water* (2005) p. Prologue xxii

Chapter 5

1. Charlotte Gerson is the daughter of Max Gerson who developed an alternative dietary cancer therapy called Gerson Therapy. Charlotte Gerson carries on his work at The Gerson Institute. www.gerson.org

2. Gamble, Foster & Kimberely Carter, *Thrive: What on Earth Will It Take?* (2011) Documentary www.thrivemovement.com

3. DAUX Acronym by Lars Gustafsson, Founder of The BodyMind Institute

4. Rodale News article by Emily Main, *9 Disturbing Side Effects of Soda* http://www.rodalenews.com/facts-about-soda

Chapter 6

1. Thomas, Lewis, *The Lives of a Cell: Notes of a Biology Watcher* (1974) p. 14 (Kindle edition)

2. Thomas, Lewis, *The Lives of a Cell: Notes of a Biology Watcher* (1974) p. 36 (Kindle edition)

3. Elliott, Aiyana, *Simply Raw: Reversing Diabetes in 30 Days* (2009)

Chapter 7

1. Peck, M. Scott, *The Road Less Traveled: A New Psychology of Love, Traditional Values and Spiritual Growth* (1978) p. 13

2. Hydrochloric Acid
http://www.bodymindbeautiful.com/hcl.html

3. Thompson, Robert, *The Calcium Lie: What Your Doctor Doesn't Know Could Kill You* (2008) p. 1

4. For more information about probiotics visit: http://www.bodyecology.com

5. Visit http://www.oneradionetwork.com with Patrick Timpone for interviews with Daniel Vitalis.
www.danielvitalis.com www.surthrival.com

6. Dangers of the microwave:
http://www.mercola.com/article/microwave/hazards2.htm

Chapter 8

1. Condron, Barbara, *The Dreamer's Dictionary* (2005) School of Metaphysics (bookstore): http://www.som.org

2. Visit http://www.oneradionetwork.com with Patrick Timpone for an interview with Dr. Rubin Naiman or visit: http://www.drnaiman.com

3. Ray Peat Ph.D. www.raypeat.com

4. Dave Asprey: Bulletproof Coffee© http://www.upgradedself.com

Chapter 9

1. Negative Ions: http://www.totalwellnessworldwide.com

2. Video: David Wolfe and Dr. Mercola discuss Multiple Sclerosis: http://www.youtube.com/watch?v=iusQ8wLIFmY

3. Ober, Sinatra, Zucker, *Earthing: The Most Important Health Discovery Ever?* (2010) pp. 58-59

Chapter 10

1. For lessons on the trivium visit: http://www.tragedyandhope.com

2. Video: Merging The Trivium Method with Non-Violent Communication: http://www.youtube.com/watch?v=XWY3jC3haR0

3. Organic Consumers http://www.organicconsumers.org

4. *Hungry for Change* (2012) Documentary, Comments by Daniel Vitalis

Chapter 11

1. Lipton, Bruce, *Spontaneous Evolution: Our Positive Future (And a Way to Get There From Here)* (2009) p. 260

2. Ruiz, Don Miguel, *The Fifth Agreement* (2010) Location 640 (Kindle edition)

3. Video interview with John Maxwell Taylor and Lilou Mace: *How to deal with negative and egoistic people.*

http://www.youtube.com/watch?v=sLHLW9Rb7FU

4. Video interview with poet David Whyte and Dr. Jeffrey Mishlove: Preserving the Soul (excerpt)

http://www.youtube.com/watch?v=Vlz3mf7jxkc

5. *Lost* Poem by David Wagoner from *Collected Poems 1956-1976* Indiana University Press.

6. Watts, Alan, *Zen Bones:On the Spirit of Zen* (1998) Audio

Chapter 12

1. *The Healthy Farmland Diet* (2013): Free Download

http://www.ucsusa.org/food_and_agriculture/solutions/expand-healthy-food-access/the-healthy-farmland-diet.html

2. Permaculture: http://www.permacultureprinciples.com

3. The Venus Project: http://www.thevenusproject.com

4. Lipton, Bruce, *The Biology of Belief* (2005) p. 95

5. Interview with David Alan Goodman, Ph. D., (August 25th, 2011), Patrick Timpone Show

http://oneradionetwork.com/geo-politics/david-goodman-ph-d-drugs-lobotomize-neuroscience-during-eisenhower-and-kennedy-years-revisited-and-reignited-today-august-25-2011/

6. Wells, S.D., Health Basics: *The 11 most toxic vaccine ingredients and their side effects.* (February 29, 2012) Learn more:

http://www.naturalnews.com/035431_vaccine_ingredients_side_effec ts_MSG.html - ixzz2oQtFiL4r

7. Humphries, Suzanne, M.D. November 17, 2011, *Smoke, Mirrors and the "Disappearance" of Polio.*
http://www.vaccinationcouncil.org/2011/11/17/smoke-mirrors-and-the-disappearance-of-polio/

8. Coase, Ronald, *"If you torture the data long enough, it will confess to anything."* Quote from Coase (economist and author) originally in the 1960's, during a talk at The University of Virginia.

9. Pollan Michael, *Playing God in the Garden,* New York Times Magazine, October 25, 1998
http://www.nytimes.com/1998/10/25/magazine/playing-god-in-the-garden.html?pagewanted=all&src=pm

10. Gatto, John Taylor, *The Prussian Reform Movement*
http://www.johntaylorgatto.com/chapters/7c.htm

11. Iserbyt, Charlotte Thomson *The Deliberate Dumbing Down of America* (1999)
For a free PDF download of the book:
http://www.deliberatedumbingdown.com

Chapter 13

1. Wachowski, Andy & Lana, *The Matrix* (1999) This statement is an adaptation from the line by Morpheus, "It is the world that has been pulled over your eyes to blind you from the truth."

2. Rajneesh, Bhagwan Shree *The Book of Wisdom Volume II* (1984) p. 30

Appendix I

1. Heap, Richard, *Consumed: Inside the Belly of the Beast* (2011)